KAMA X...

A sex guide with 3D holog...

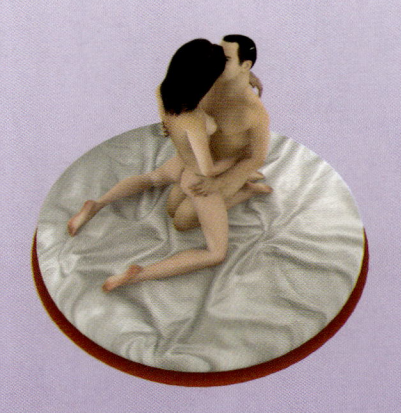

69 interactive positions with free apps

Published by Xcite Books Ltd – 2013

ISBN 9781909335257

Copyright © Xcite Books 2013

The right of Xcite Books to be identified as the author of this work has been asserted by them in accordance with the Copyright, Designs and Patents Act 1988.

All rights reserved. No part of this book may be copied, or transmitted in any form or by any means, electronic, electrostatic, magnetic tape, mechanical, photocopying, recording or otherwise, without the written permission of the publishers:

Xcite Books, Suite 11769, 2nd Floor, 145-157 St John Street, London EC1V 4PY

ABOUT THE KAMA XCITRA

The Kama Sutra is one of the oldest sex manuals in existence, originally written by Mallinaga Vatsayana, an Indian sage, over 2000 years ago. Today, the book is best known for its lavish descriptions of sex positions, from the simple to the almost impossibly athletic.

Until now, some of the more challenging positions have left readers a little baffled. However, the Kama Xcitra adds an interactive twist, letting you get closer to the action than ever before as you explore these positions from every angle, using the smartphone or tablet app which accompanies this book to bring the illustrations to life in 3D.

The positions here do not have to be used in sequence, as the original text suggested; you can try several in one session, or stick to only one, depending on your mood. Each is graded for its difficulty, from 1 to 3, as some require you to have more stamina and suppleness than others, and not all may be suitable if you have a bad back, or if one partner is much bigger or heavier than the other.

●○○ Easy – suitable for everyone
●●○ Medium – takes the passion up a level
●●● Expert – handle with care

Unlike other versions of the guide, we let you know what each position is best for. You will quickly find your favourites, whether you're looking for sex that is fast or slow, gentle or intense.

DOWNLOADING THE FREE APP

Welcome to the first truly interactive Kama Xcitra.

Now that you have the book bring the Kama Xcitra alive and into the 21st Century by downloading and using the free smartphone or tablet apps that accompany the book. Here's how:

To download the free app, go to the Kama Xcitra's website at **www.kamaxcitra.com**; here is where you will find detailed instructions on the app and how to download it.

Using the Kama Xcitra smartphone or tablet app:

- Open the app
- You will then be presented with all the Kama Xcitra positions
- Click on the position which corresponds with the one you are viewing in the book
- Once the main screen has loaded, you will see two buttons, one in the top left and top right hand corners which look like this respectively:
- These two buttons allow you to access the functionality menu
- Click on the button again and this hides the menu.
- Have a play with the functionality yourself. Alternatively, refer to the **www.kamaxcitra.com** website or click on the help button inside the functionality menu to find out more about the app and what it can do

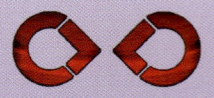

- So with the app running, point the smartphone or tablet camera at the couple on the page demonstrating the sexual position that you want to 'pop up' in 3D. We've included an onscreen positioning marker to help you

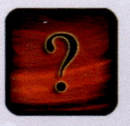

- Make sure that the camera lens of your smartphone or tablet is not covered in any way and also make sure that the illustration in the book and its border are all in camera shot

- Hey presto! The image at which you are pointing your smartphone or tablet computer will suddenly pop up to become a 3D image on your smartphone or tablet screen

- Take some time to experiment. Try moving your smartphone or tablet computer around and with the camera lens still pointed at the illustration in the book you can see around and over the couple so as to appreciate the finer details of the sexual position. You can also rotate the book to achieve the same effect.

- Alternatively, keep your smartphone or tablet computer still and swipe left/right to trigger rotation and the 3D image will start to spin slowly before your eyes

- You cannot use the app without the book but, let's face it, it will be almost impossible to test out one of these sexual positions while holding your smartphone or tablet computer over the Kama Xcitra book! So, if you want to keep the 3D image on your screen while you get into position then the image can be frozen to enable you to refer to it while you get, ahem, cracking.

And there you have it. Have fun and let us know what you think about it.

1. THE BOSTON BRUTE

A derivative of The Union of the Monkey, this position requires a great deal of stability. The woman lies on her back and raises her legs in the air while the man sits on her thighs with his back and bends his penis back down towards her vagina. He controls the up and down movement while she can provide additional gyration. The thrill comes from the unusual angle of penetration.

DIFFICULTY
● ● ●

Best for: creative couples, and men who have an exceptionally flexible penis

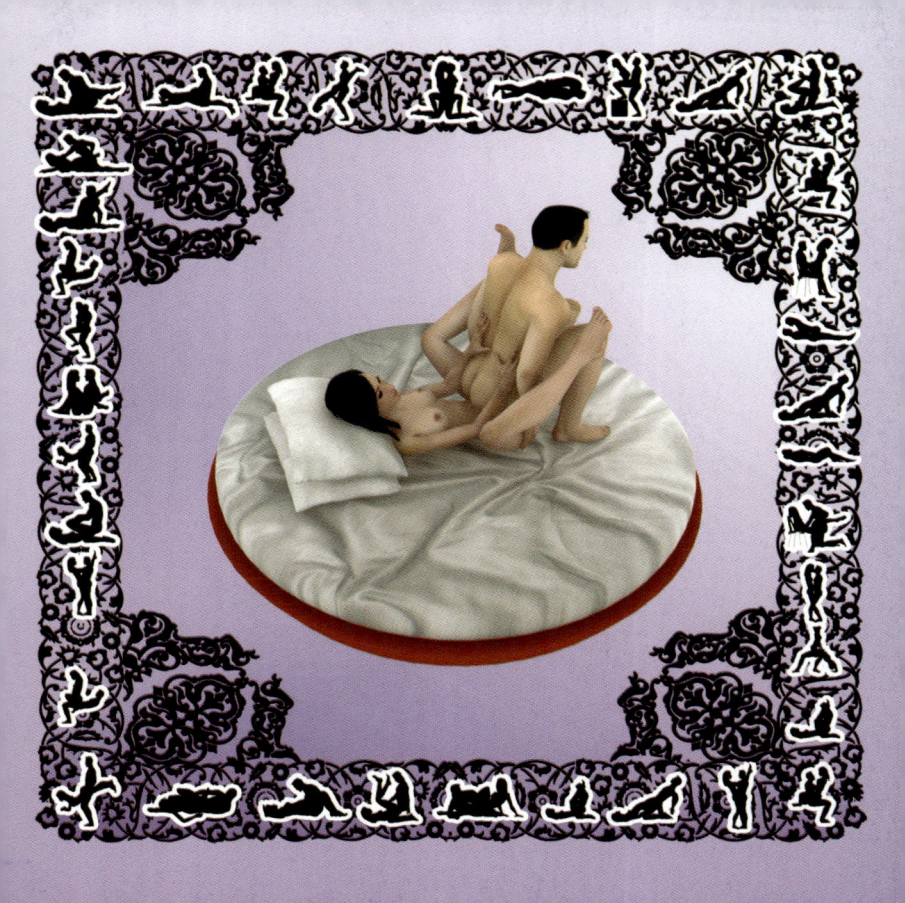

2. THE LOVE SEAT

Also known as the Union of the Scorpion. The woman lies back on the man with her legs spread behind or in front of her, depending on flexibility. This position provides a great deal of intimate contact and leaves the man with free access to all the woman's zones of pleasure, from breasts to clitoris.

DIFFICULTY
● ● ○

Best for: maximum body contact between lovers

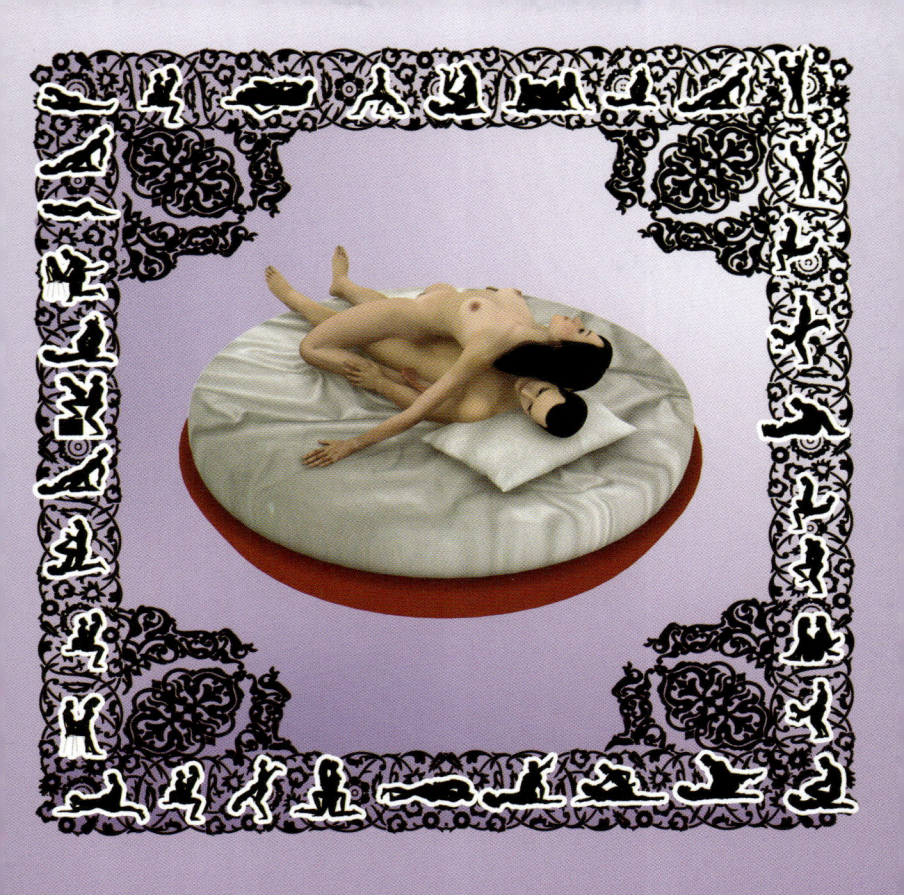

3. THE COW GIRL

Very similar to the Position of Andromache, where the woman is also on top. However, here the woman is in a crouching position as opposed to kneeling over the man. This allows her to exert far more control and power, setting the rhythm of movements as she shifts up and down on his penis.

DIFFICULTY

●○○

Best for: couples who like to entertain fantasies of female domination

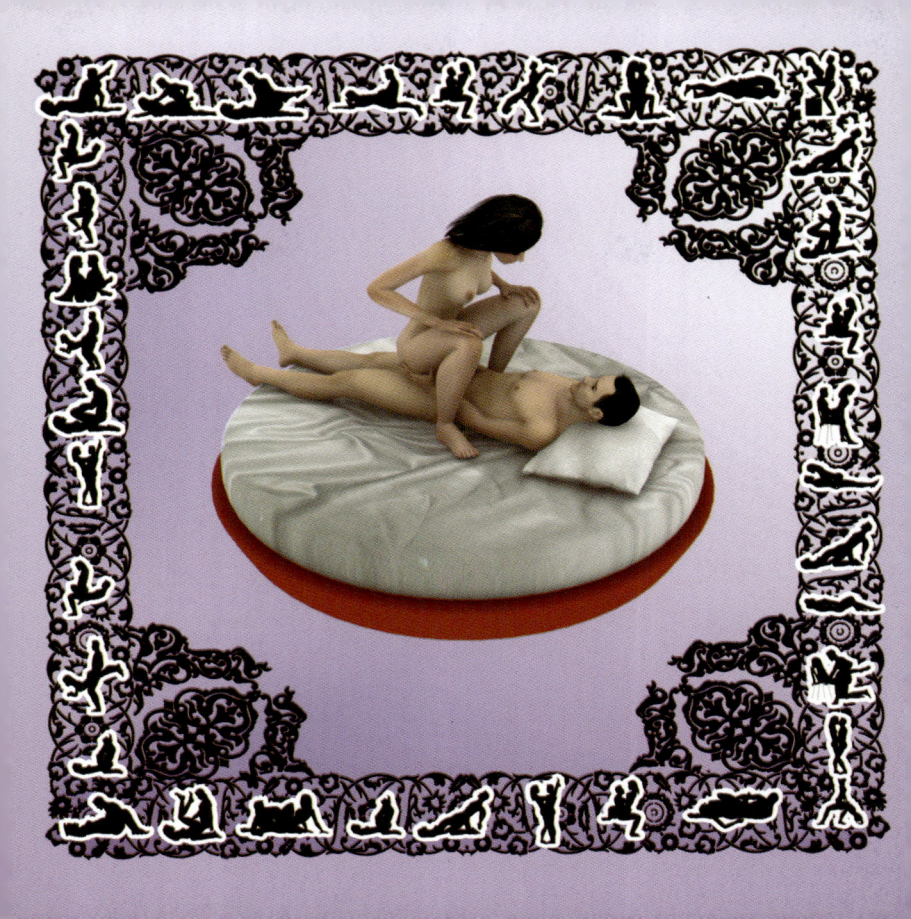

4. THE OCTOPUS

The man sits with his legs out in front of him, supporting himself with his arms. The woman sits in his lap, facing him, with her legs spread in front of her, also using her arms to hold herself up. This allows the woman to rock her pelvis in a wide variety of motions in order to achieve a mutual climax.

DIFFICULTY
● ● ●

Best for: couples with strong arm and shoulder muscles

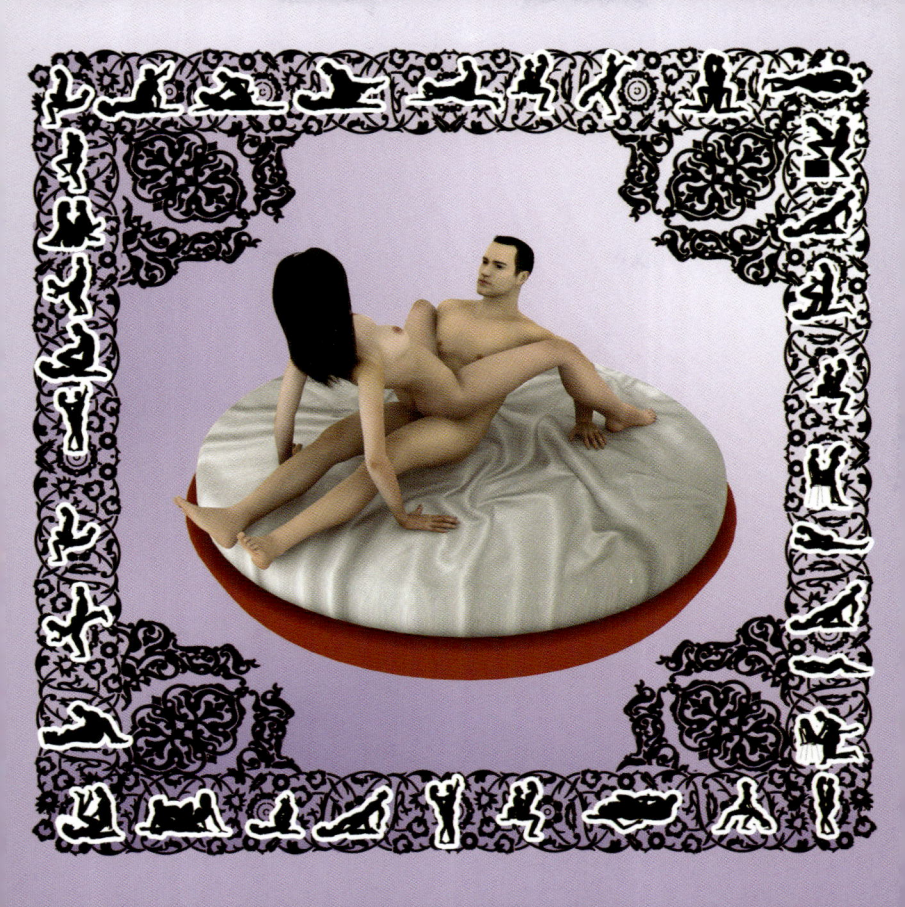

5. THE BUCKING BRONCO

The man sits with his legs stretched out in front of him and supported by his hands. The woman does the same, facing him, but with her legs hooked over his shoulders. This not only allows her to control the speed and range of her movements but also allows the man to provide the ultimate ride.

DIFFICULTY
● ● ●

Best for: deep penetration

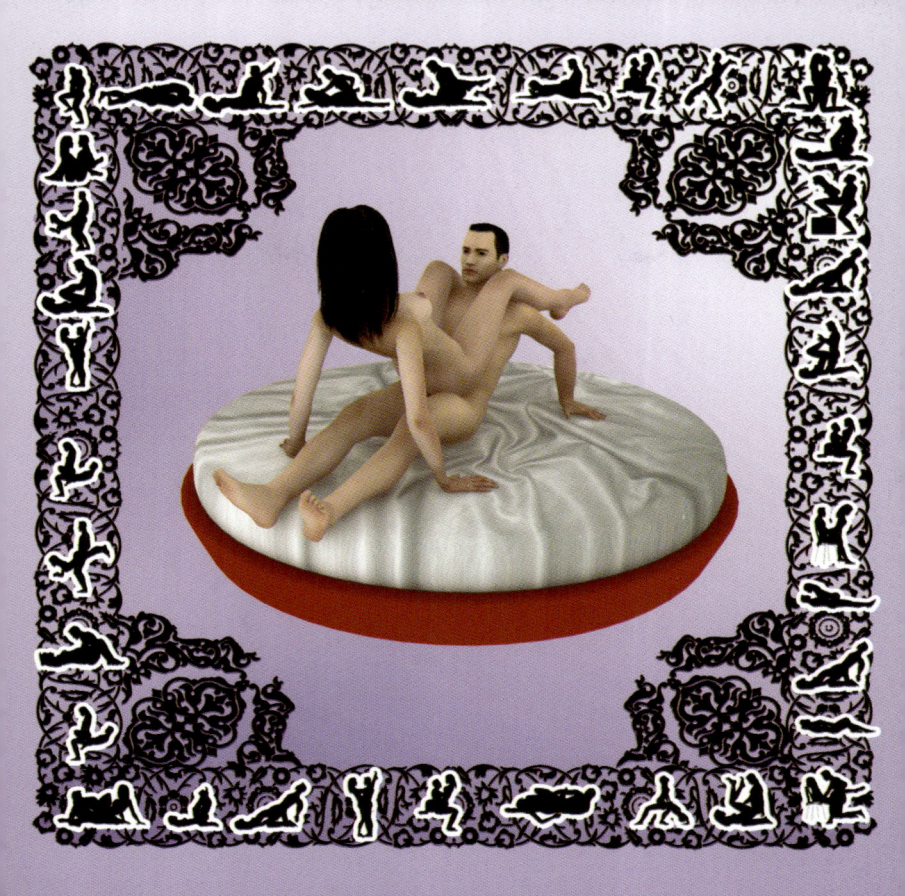

6. THE INVERTED MISSIONARY

The Position of Andromache, and the starting point for the Cow Girl. The man lies on his back and the woman positions herself in a squatting position above him. This allows her to take charge of the rhythm and depth of the thrusts, while offering the man free access to her key pleasure spots.

DIFFICULTY

● ○ ○

Best for: her orgasm, as she controls the experience

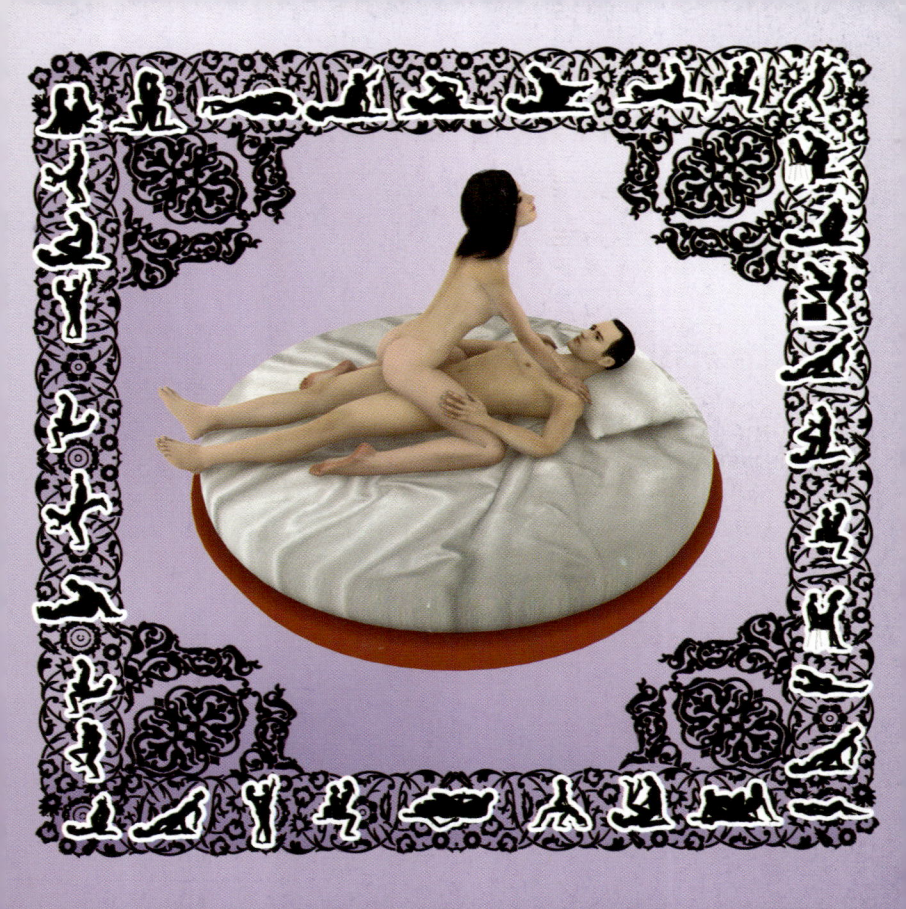

7. THE EDGE OF HEAVEN

Also known as the Union of the Magpie, this position involves the man sitting on the edge of the bed. The woman sits in his lap, facing him, with her legs astride his body. This allows for greater penetration and fairly vigorous movement.

DIFFICULTY

● ○ ○

Best for: couples where the woman is heavier, as bed and man combine to support her weight

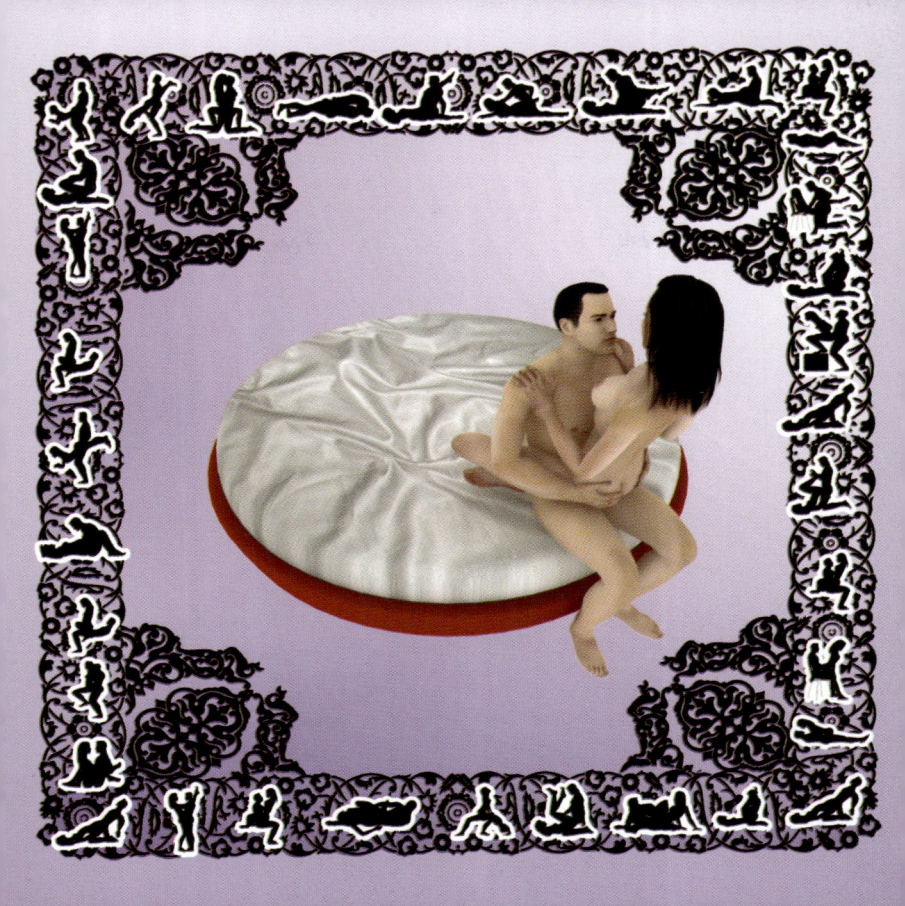

8. THE CHAMPAGNE ROOM

The Posture of Balance. The man sits on the edge of the bed and the woman sits down on his thighs, facing away from him. If the woman spreads her legs wide enough she can use the man's knees to obtain the position of perfect balance. Lacks the intimacy of the Union of the Magpie, as in this position there is no possibility of eye contact.

DIFFICULTY

● ● ○

Best for: unrestricted access to the woman's breasts and clitoris

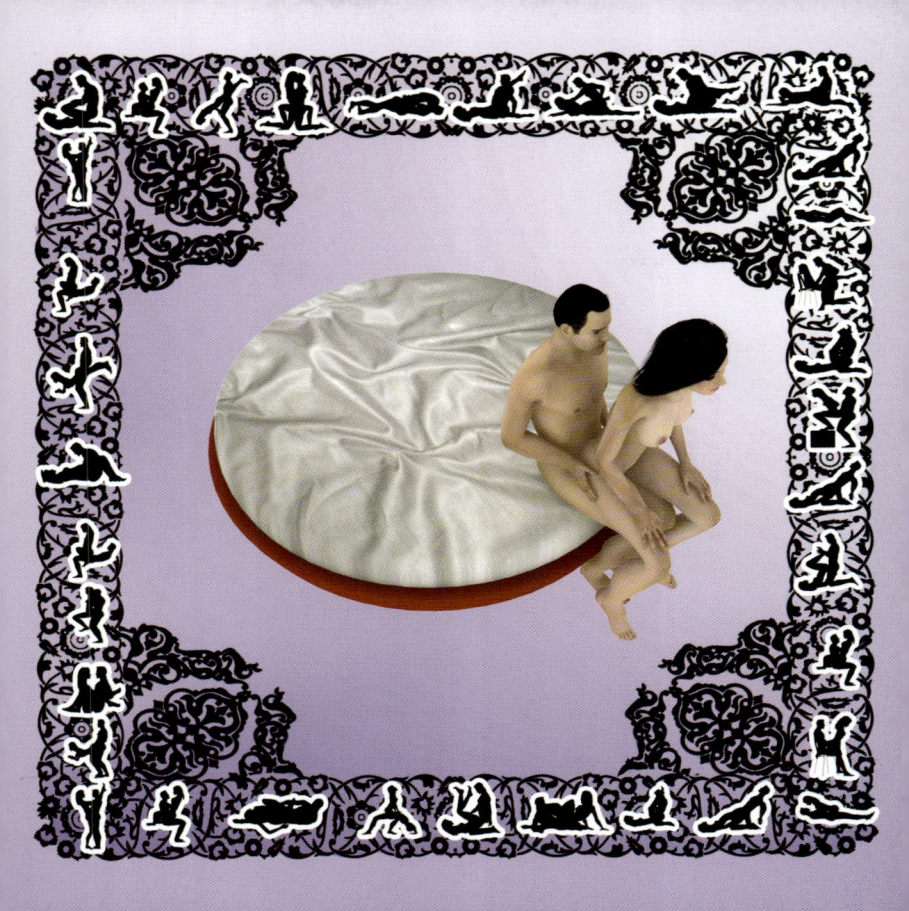

9. THE CHAIR

The man sits on a chair with his partner on his lap and facing away from him, in a kneeling position with her legs off the floor. She then uses the strength in her legs to make an up-and-down bouncing movement, while he caresses her clitoris and breasts. If the woman leans forward, it will allow for easier penetration.

DIFFICULTY
●●●

Best for: men with back problems, as the chair back offers extra support

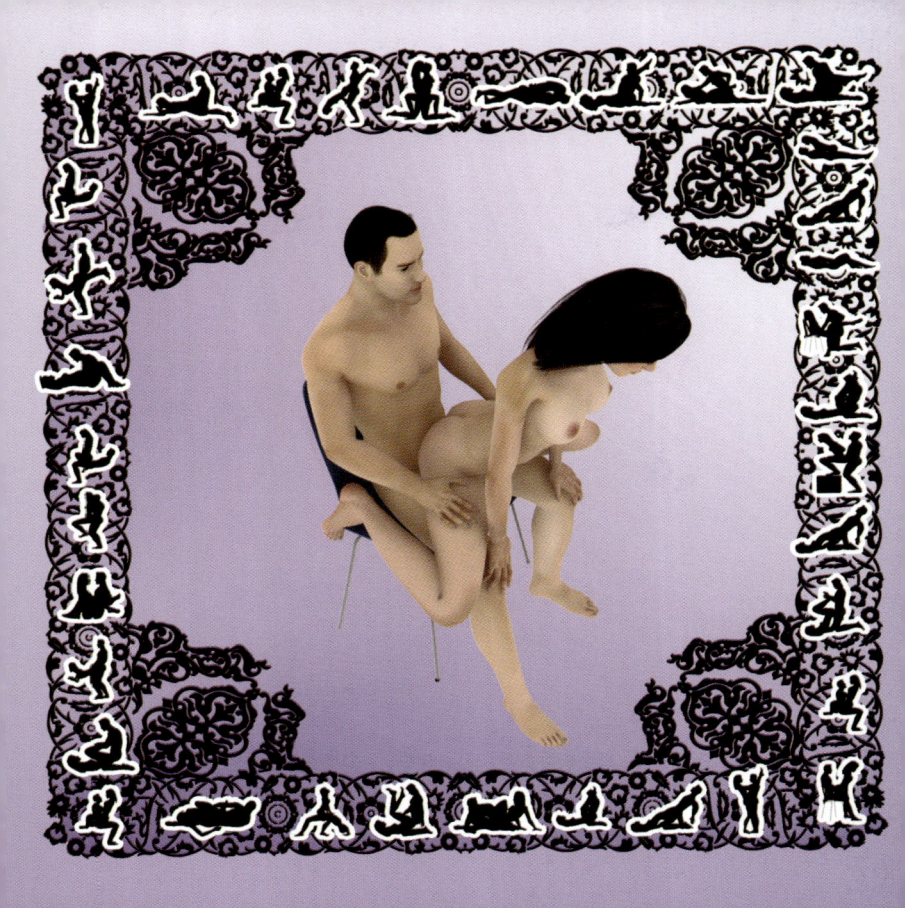

10. THE BIG GAME

For the more subservient amongst you, and perfectly designed for the football fanatic. Experience the highs of two sports at the same time, as the man can watch the big game on TV while the woman performs oral sex on him. If the results are good, the after-match entertainment may well be worth putting in all the work; if not, a considerate lover will return the favour anyway.

DIFFICULTY

● ○ ○

Best for: women with submissive fantasies

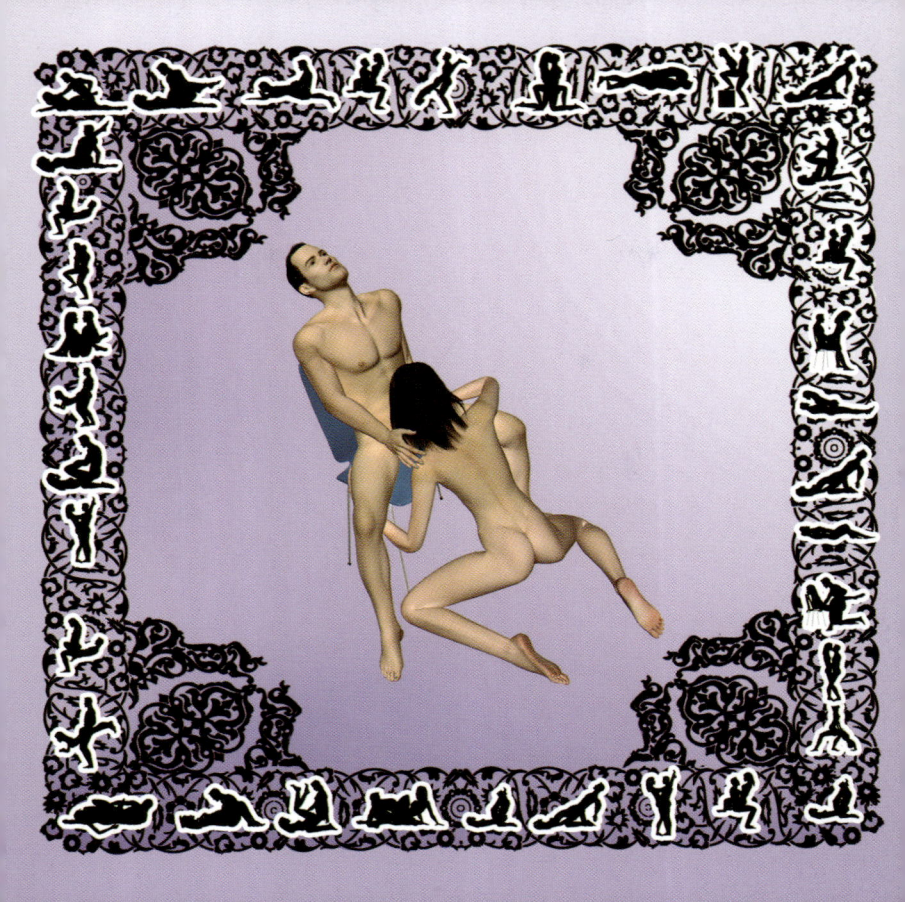

11. RIDE THE SLIDE

This position gives the woman the ultimate control of both direction and depth. The man lies on his back, and the woman lies on top of him with her legs spread wide. While he penetrates her, she begins to slide up and down his body, rubbing and teasing. In this position, the man may be surprised by how much tighter she feels.

DIFFICULTY

●○○

Best for: those men who like to be tightly gripped by their lover's vagina

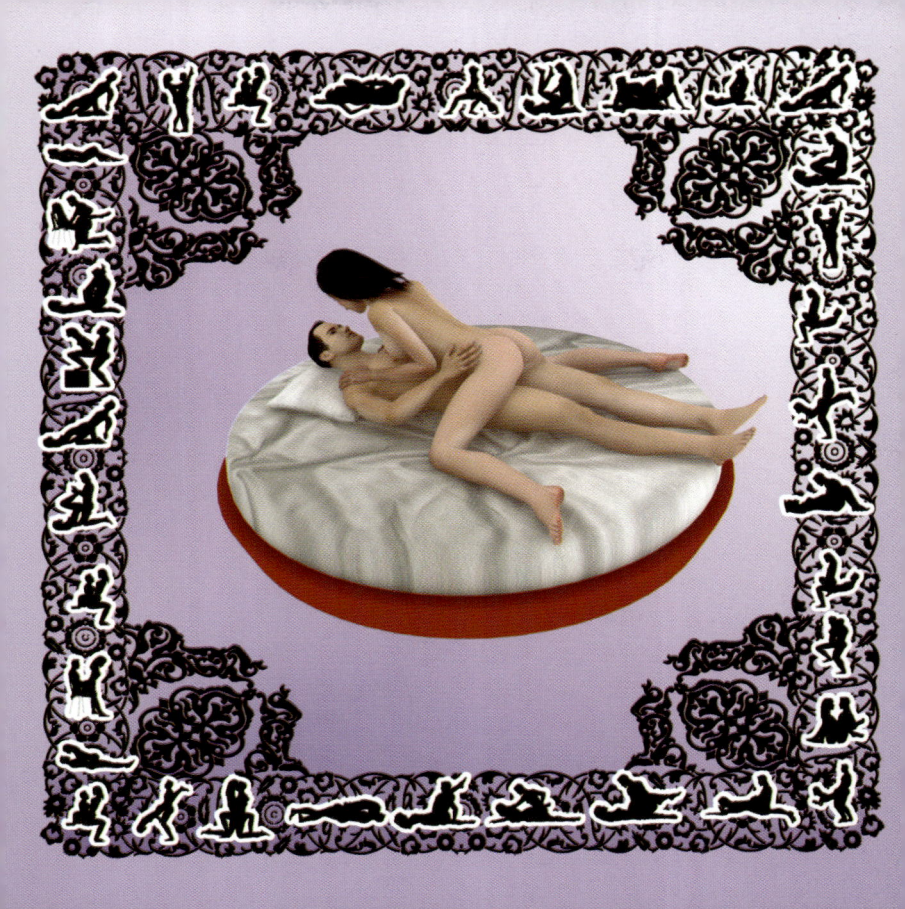

12. THE LAZY BOY

The man creates a chair with his body for the woman to recline into. She lies in the chair with her legs spread to control the movement. This allows the woman to play with both her clitoris and the man's testicles. It also offers him a tantalizing view and the freedom to access it with his hands.

DIFFICULTY

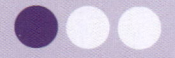

● ○ ○

Best for: transitioning from one position to another, as it's easy for him to roll her into a new position

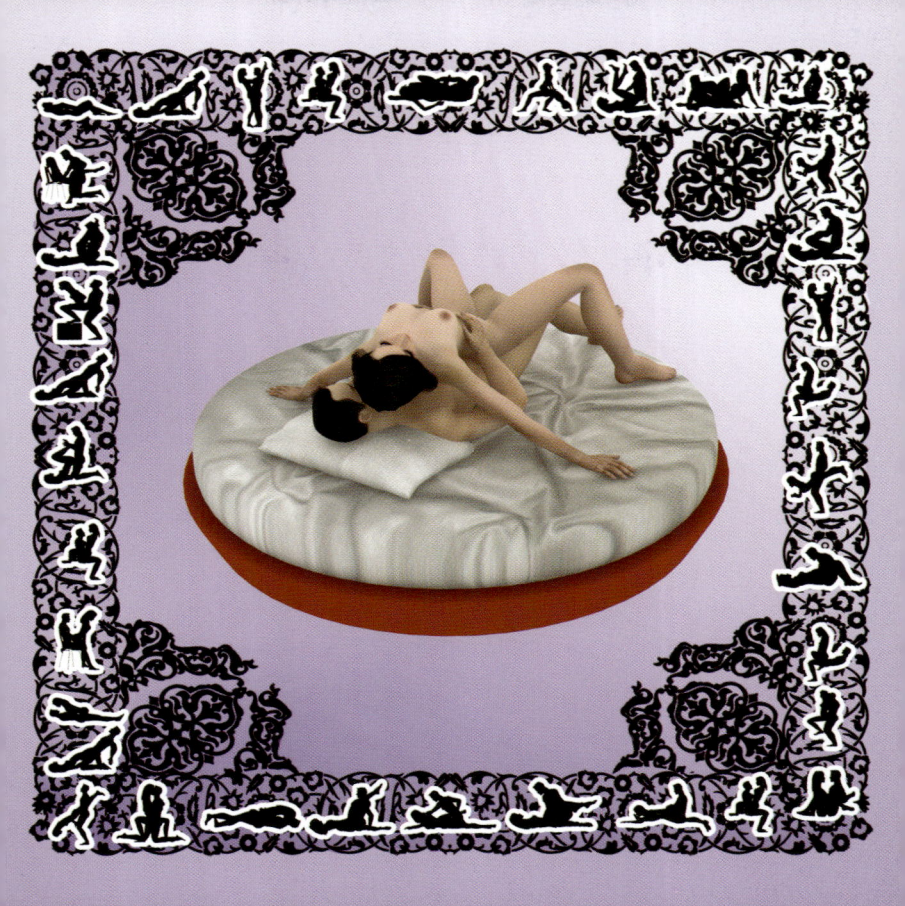

13. THE JOYSTICK

The man lies back with the woman kneeling astride him whilst facing away from him, in a reverse Cow Girl position. The woman now dictates all movement. It's one of the most exciting positions for her, as she can take mesmerising control of the pleasure both received and given, while the man can play with all her most intimate places.

DIFFICULTY

●●○

Best for: women who like to be on top – in all senses!

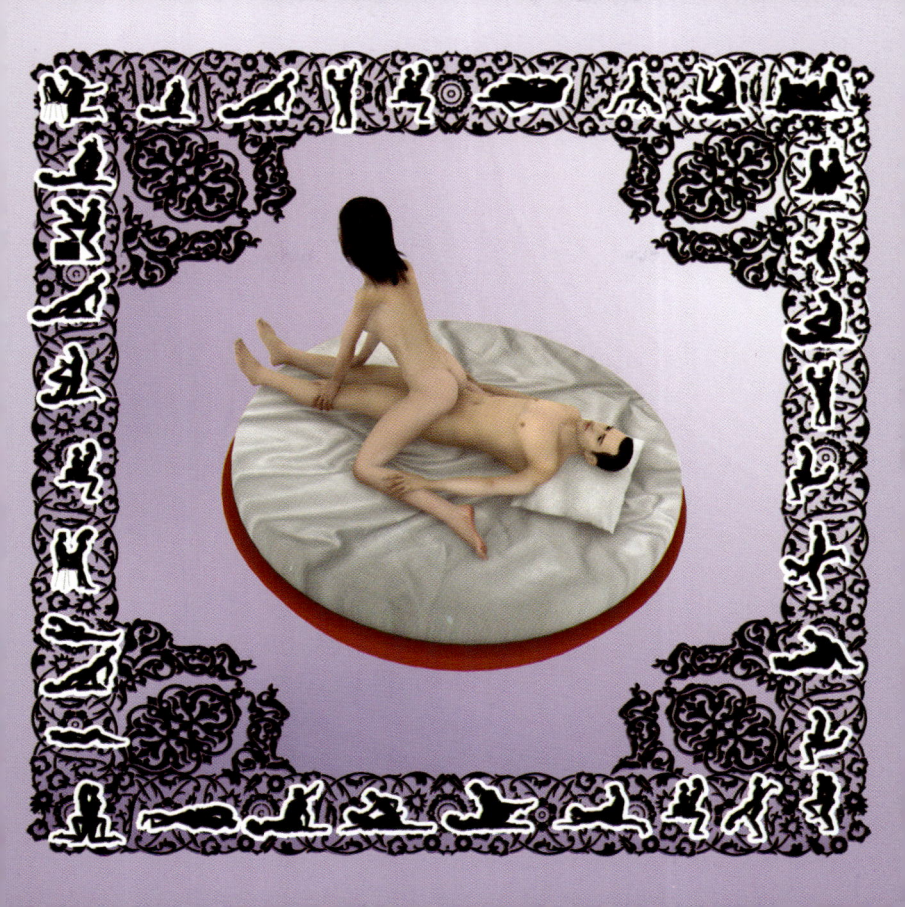

14. THE HALF LOTUS

The Union of the Butterfly, where the woman sits in the man's lap facing him, both with their legs outstretched. Less demanding than the full Lotus, in which the man's legs are crossed and the woman's are wrapped round his waist. The position allows for full facial contact whilst both partners play a role in the action. However, it does take the hands out of the picture and requires a little athleticism.

DIFFICULTY
●●○

Best for: whispering endearments to each other while you make love

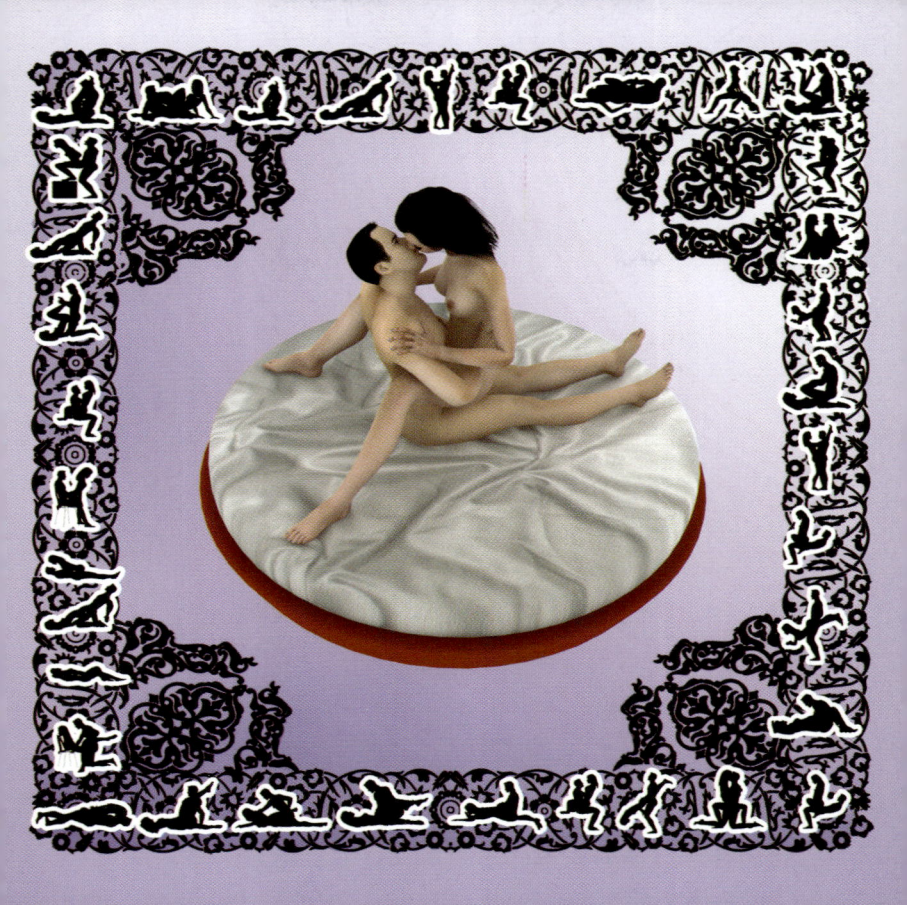

15. THE LOVE MACHINE

Similar to the Union of the Octopus, with the man adopting a fairly standard position on top of his lover. This has the advantage of being comfortable for both the man and woman and leaves their hands mostly free to take part in the activity, while she can raise her legs to offer more depth of penetration.

DIFFICULTY
● ○ ○

Best for: beginners, and those who love the missionary position

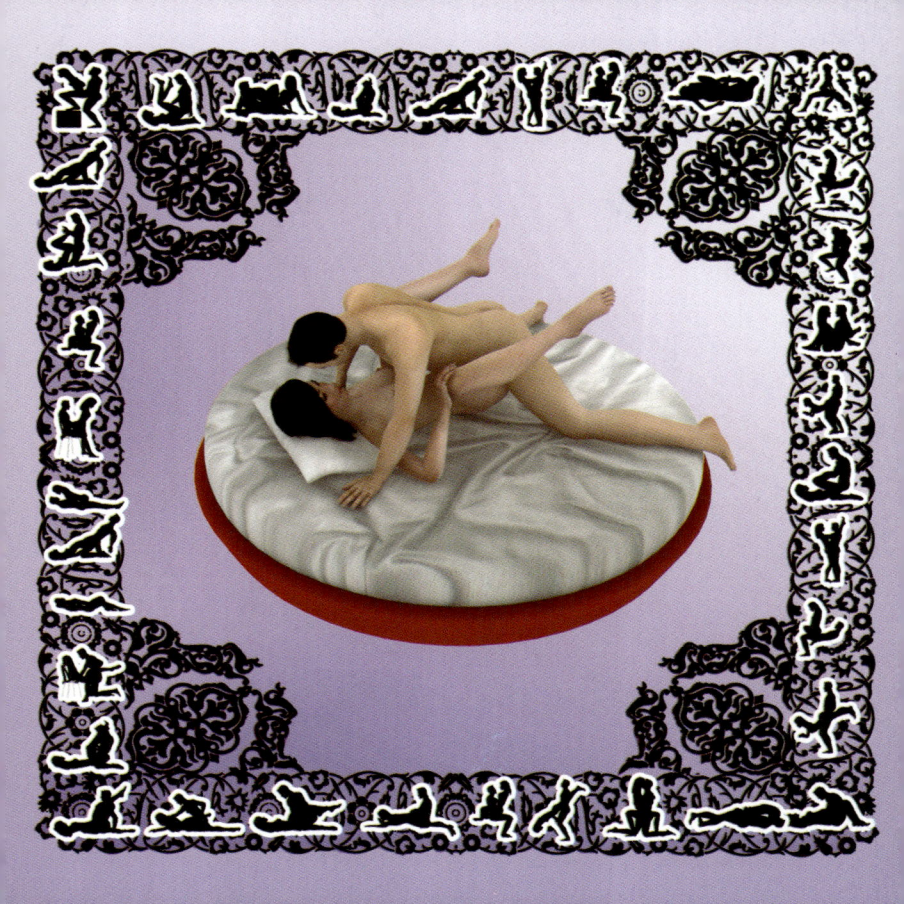

16. THE TORRID TRIANGLE

Initially, this would appear to be the standard missionary position. However, the woman's bent legs allow her to push up with her pelvis, raising the man, who supports most of his own weight. An interesting twist on vanilla lovemaking, with the woman underneath but still able to dictate the pace.

DIFFICULTY

● ○ ○

Best for: transitioning from the missionary position to something a little more adventurous

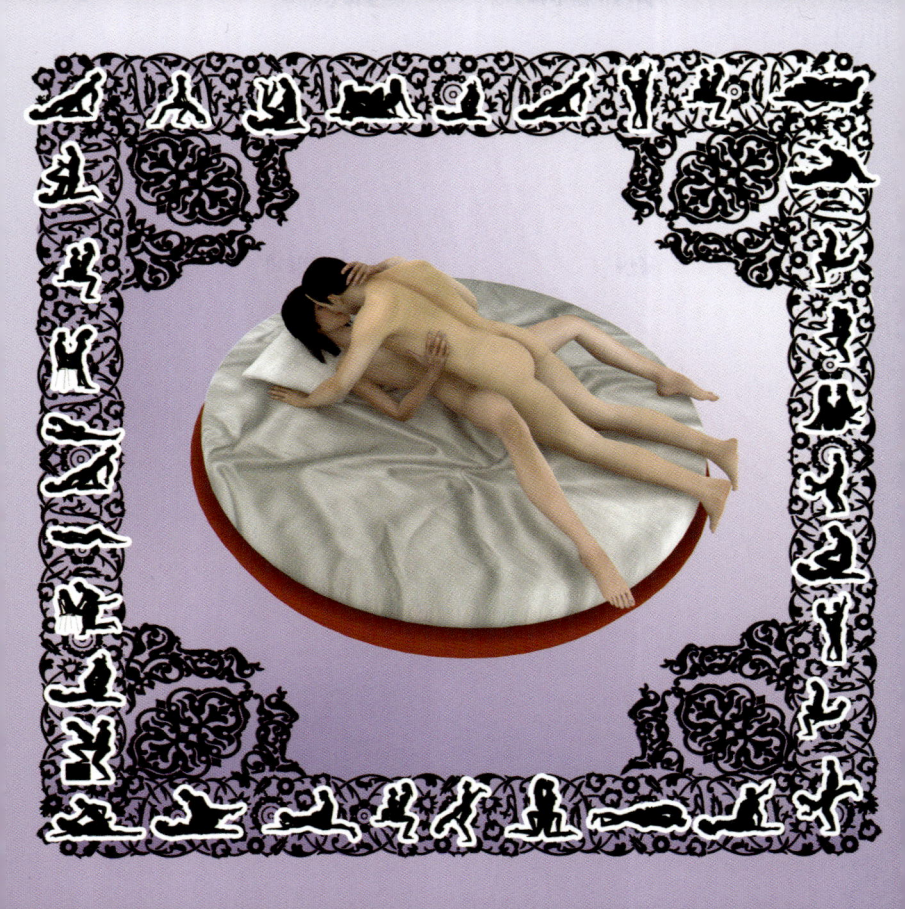

17. THE SPEED BUMP

Also known as the Union of the Elephant. The man lies on top of the woman who is facing down on the bed, raising herself up on her elbows. His legs between the woman's, he enters from the rear. This provides maximum connection with the G-spot and also allows the woman to squeeze her thighs together, increasing pressure on his penis.

DIFFICULTY
● ● ○

Best for: G-spot stimulation

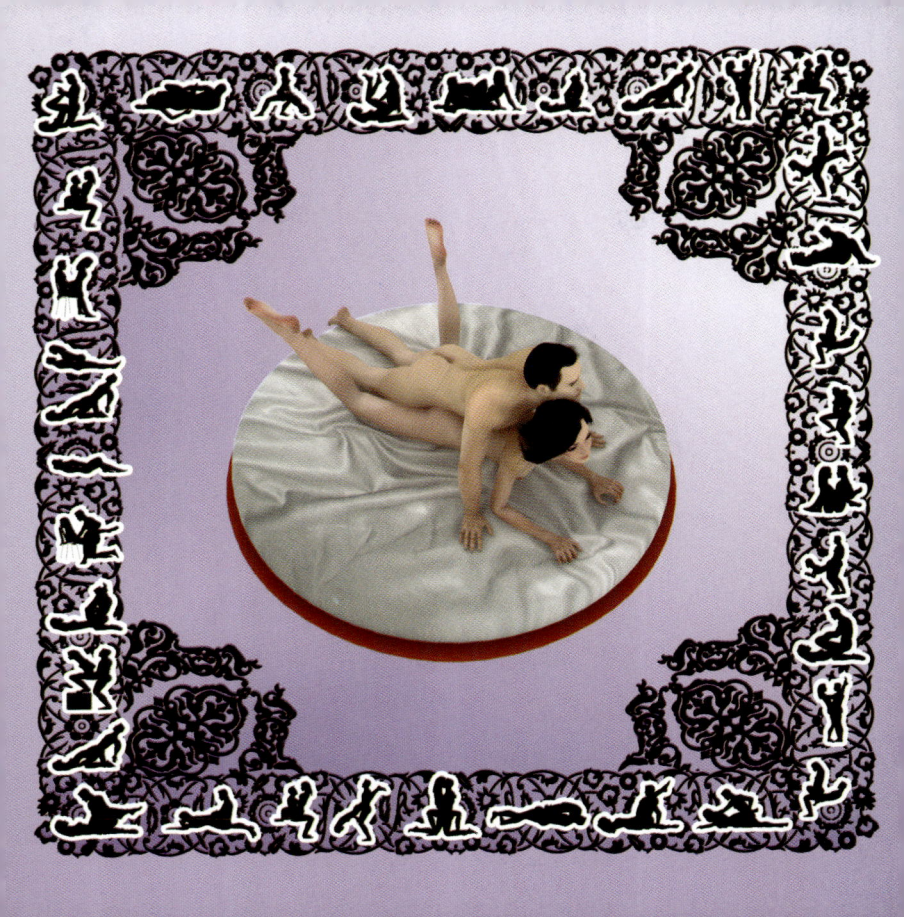

18. THE TIGHT SQUEEZE

The woman lies face down with her legs clenched tight. The man lies on top and enters from behind. The woman may cross her legs for an even tighter grip on his penis. This position allows her to feel every inch of him inside her.

DIFFICULTY

● ● ○

Best for: women who've practised their Kegel exercises – or want to, while the man is inside them

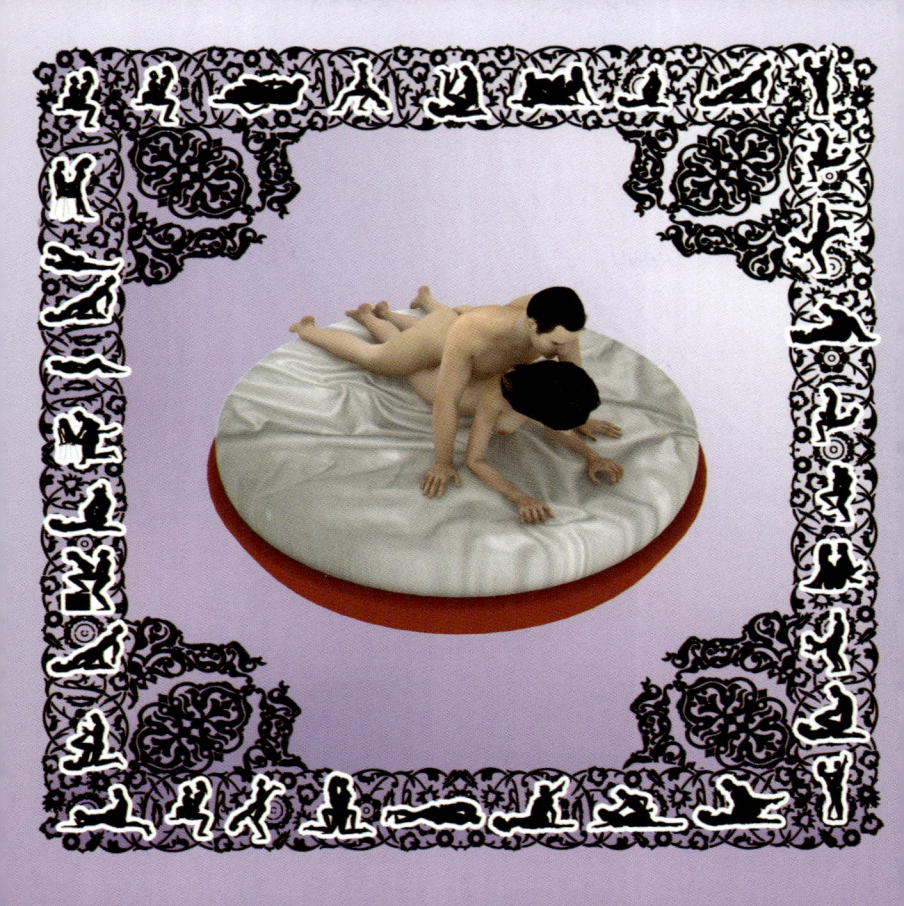

19. HIT THE SPOT

Another G-Spot speciality position, and one which can be easily transitioned into from the Speed Bump or the Tight Squeeze. With the legs bent and squeezed together, the woman can increase the man's experience significantly. With practice, she can guide him to the desired spot with ease, resulting in supreme ecstasy.

DIFFICULTY

● ● ○

Best for: the ultimate in G-spot stimulation

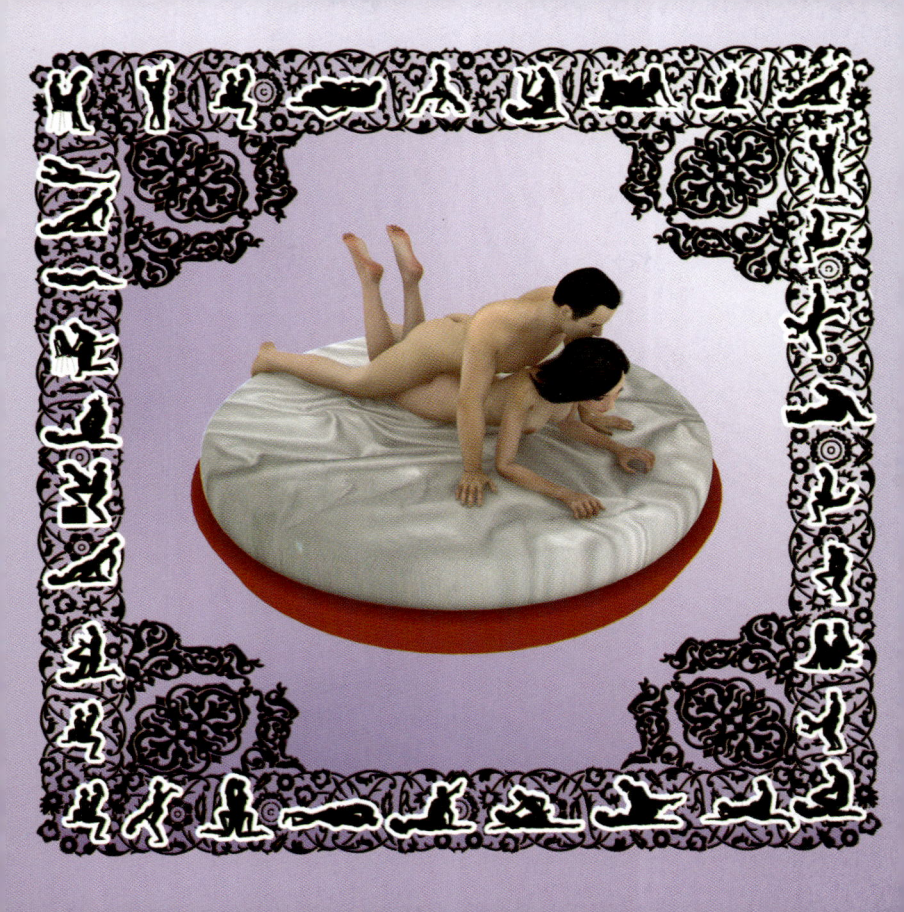

20. FORBIDDEN FRUIT

Enables a man to take his woman to the peaks of pleasure with both tongue and fingers. The woman raises her legs to provide unrestricted access to her vulva and clitoris. Performed correctly, this position will leave the man in complete control and the woman happy that he is.

DIFFICULTY

●●○

Best for: those men who like to eat out

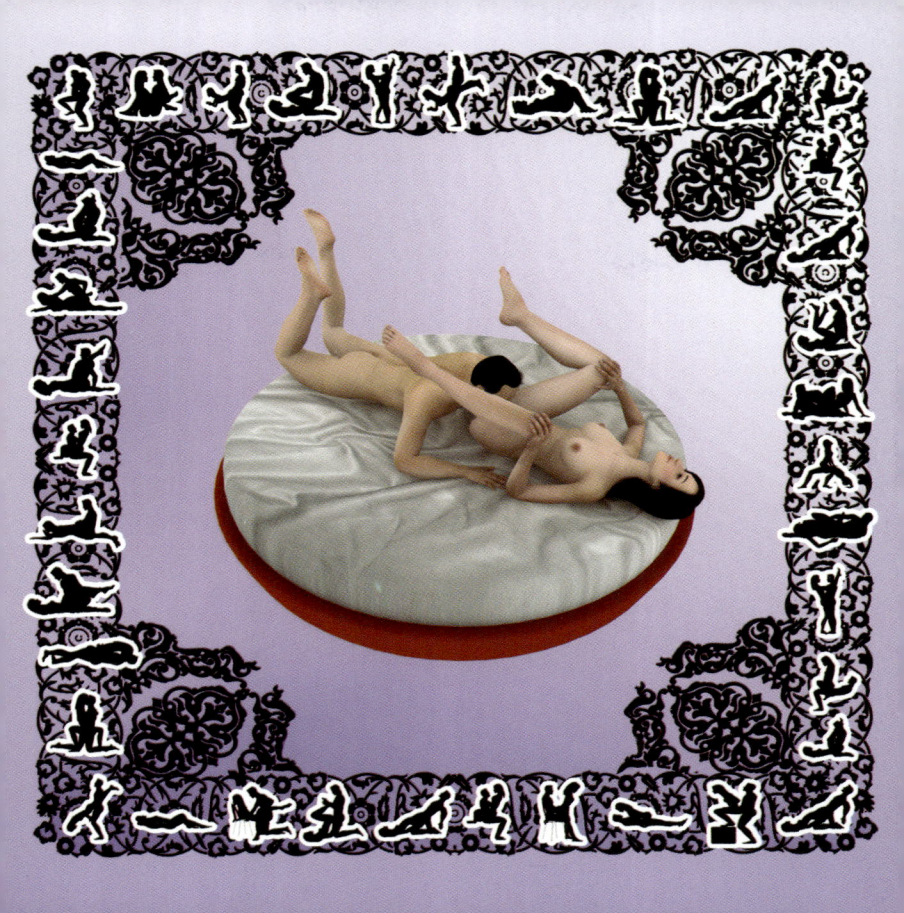

21. THE SUPPORTED DOGGY STRETCH

The woman gets on the bed, kneeling on all fours. With the man kneeling behind her, he raises her by the hips, allowing her to wrap her legs around his thighs for additional support. This allows for good penetration, but can place pressure on the woman's shoulders if performed for an extended period.

DIFFICULTY

● ● ●

Best for: couples where the woman has good upper body strength

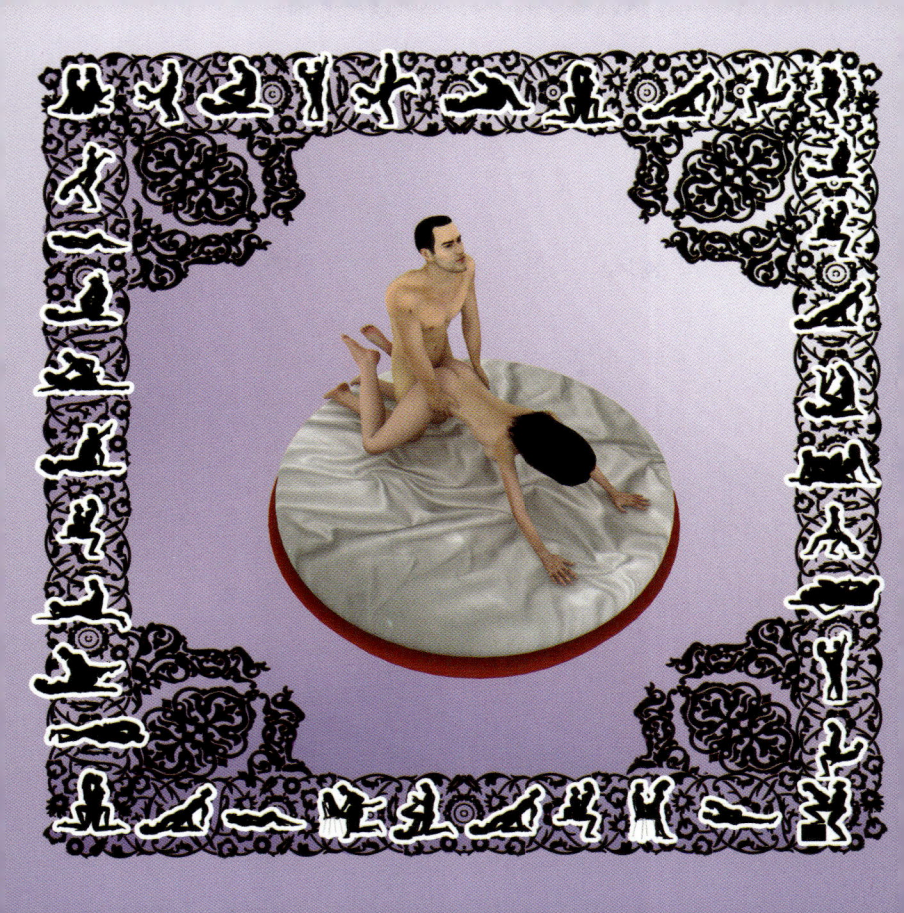

22. THE WHEELBARROW

For the more dominant and energetic, this relative of the Doggy Stretch can be quite demanding for the woman. She takes the weight on her arms and the man raises her by her hips, supporting her weight on his thighs. This allows the man to control the motion with both his body and his hands as he thrusts into her. If the man is significantly taller than the woman, she can rest on a pillow or two to make entry easier.

DIFFICULTY
● ● ●

Best for: quickie sex, as this position can be difficult to maintain for any length of time

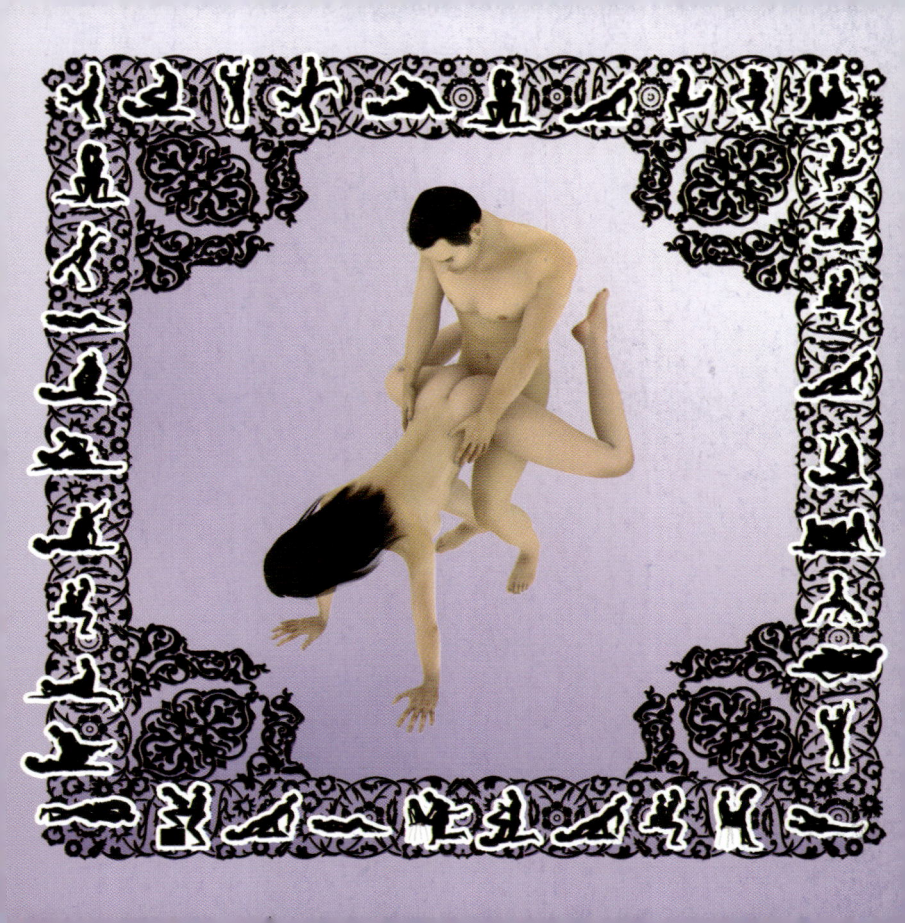

23. IRONING THE CRACKS

Also known as The Union of the Cow, this position, in which the woman's body is supported by a chair and the man kneels behind her, provides for extremely good stimulation of the vaginal walls, and especially the G-Spot. It also allows both partners to stimulate each other's genitals, and the lack of face-to-face contact means they can fantasise about being with someone other than their partner, if they wish.

DIFFICULTY

● ● ○

Best for: those who dream of a secret lover

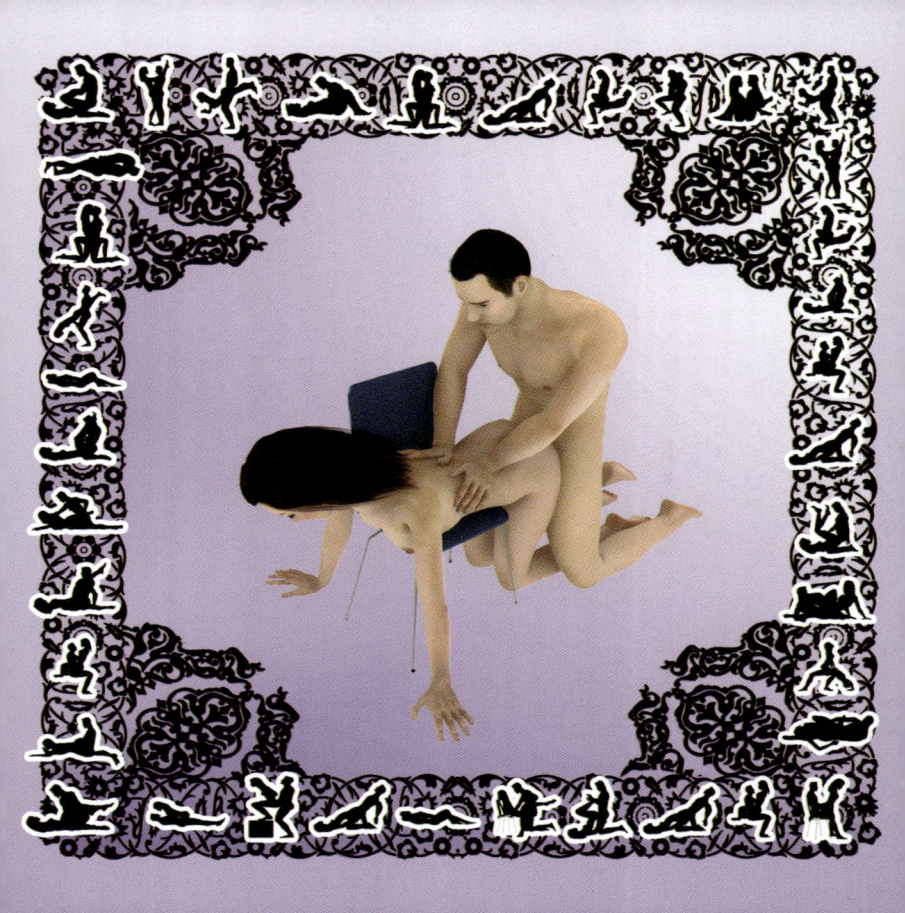

24. THE G-SPOT GIGGY

With the woman on all fours, the man enters her from behind. He is now able to control things with his hands on her hips. In this position, the penis should stroke the G-spot, providing the most exquisite of orgasms. Though some women dislike the lack of intimacy in being taken from behind, this classic position should be in every couples' repertoire.

DIFFICULTY

● ○ ○

Best for: men who like to be in charge

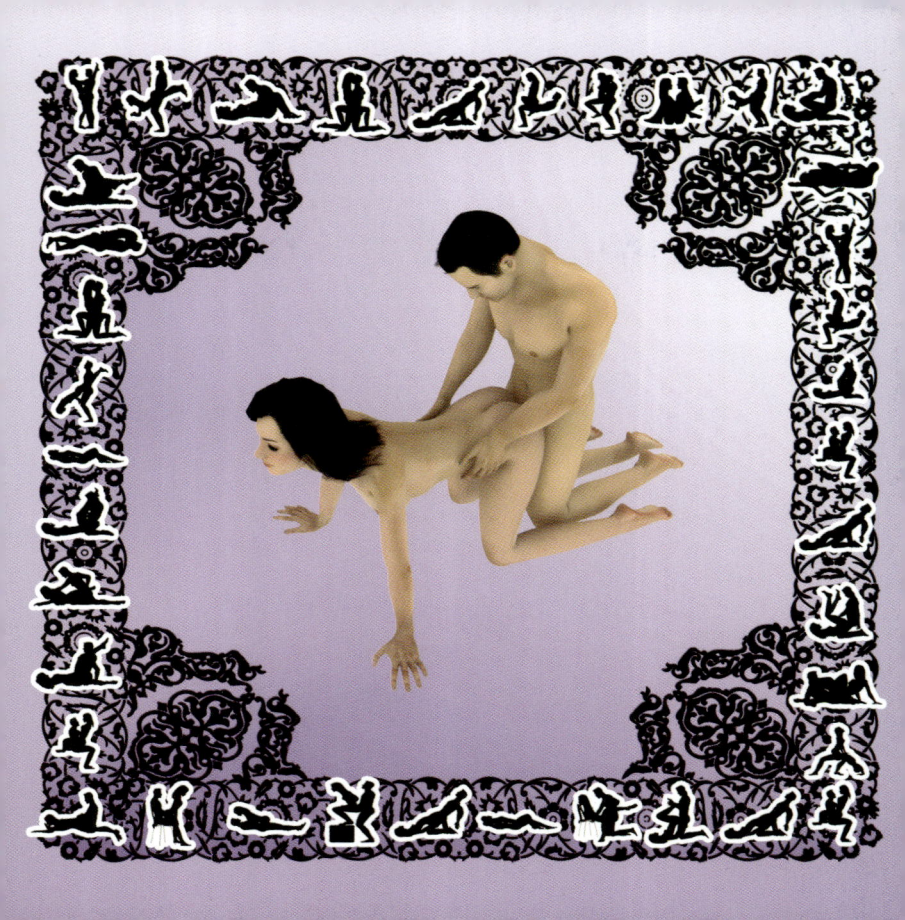

25. THE SPOONING POSITION

Lie curled up side by side with the woman in the man's arms. She should push back with her pelvis. Wrapping her upper leg around the man will allow him to enter with more ease. This is an affectionate position: the ability it allows to play with the woman's breasts and clitoris makes up for any lack of eye contact.

DIFFICULTY

●○○

Best for: pregnant women, as no pressure is placed on the stomach

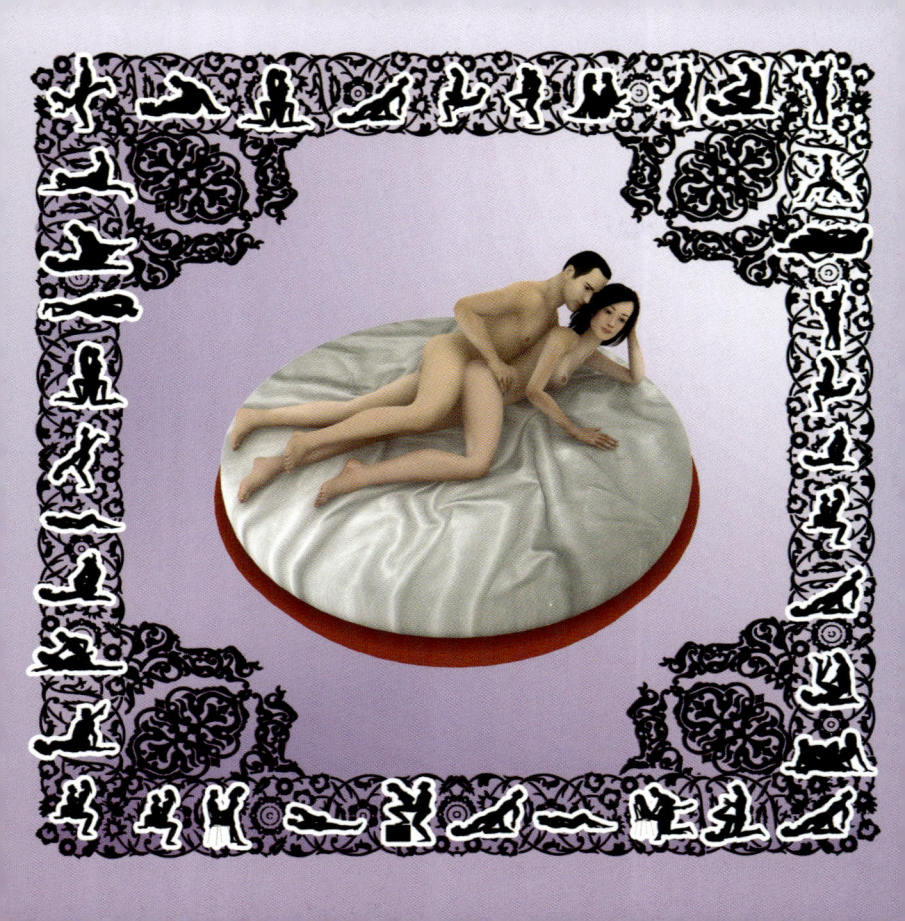

26. THE TWINING

The man lies behind the woman and enters her from behind. He straddles her with his thigh, so their bodies are twined together. By raising and lowering her leg, he can vary the depth of his penetration. This position is related to Splitting the Bamboo, but requires less energy and stamina.

DIFFICULTY

● ● ○

Best for: feeling the closeness of your lover's body against yours

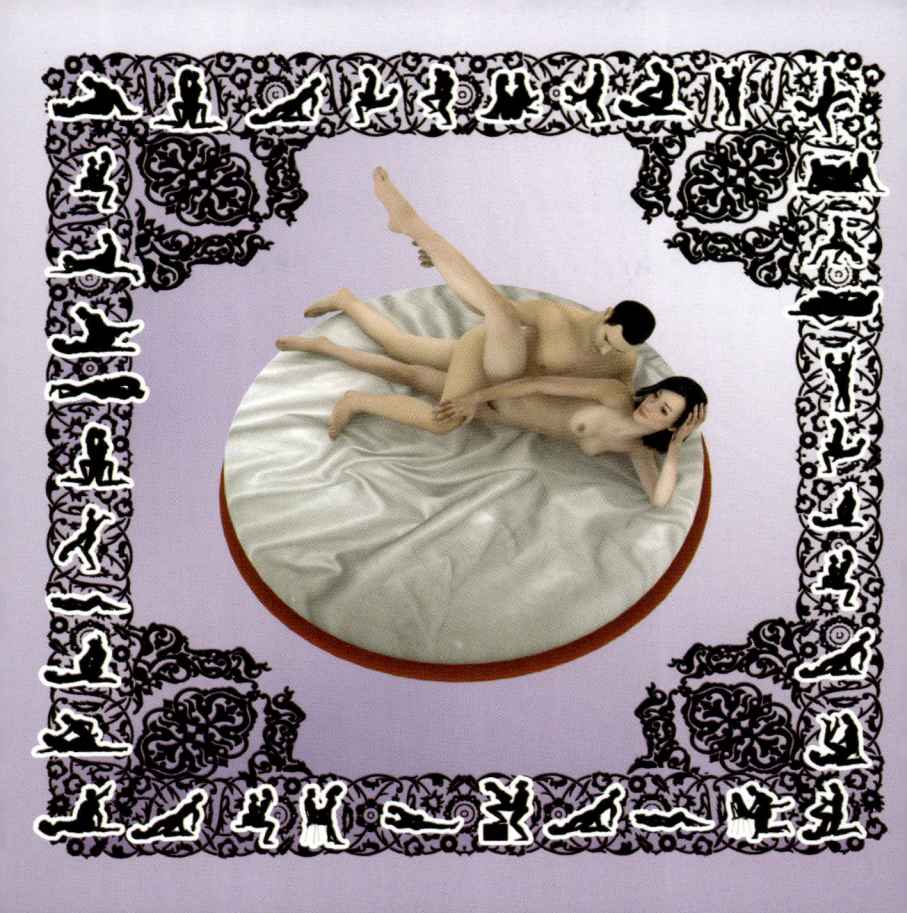

27. THE HOOK

Also known as the Posture of the Star. The woman lies on her back, with one leg bent up and the other lying flat on the ground. The man sits between her legs and pushes a leg under her bottom to raise her hip. This position allows each partner a free hand for exploration and also provides a different type of stimulation to the woman.

DIFFICULTY
● ● ●

Best for: stroking, touching and teasing during penetration

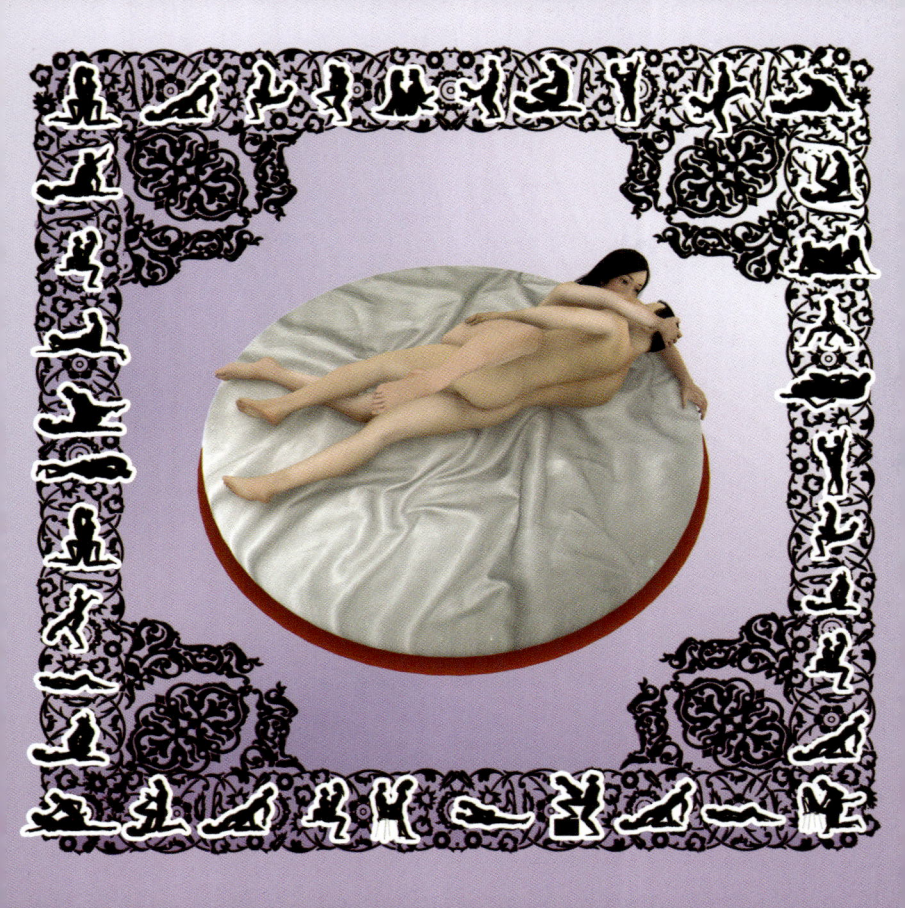

28. THE COLUMN

With both partners standing, and the woman in front with her back to the man, they interlock arms for stability. While she arches her back, he enters from behind. Deeper penetration can be obtained if the woman leans forward against a wall or a table for support, which will also help to maintain balance.

DIFFICULTY

● ● ○

Best for: those whose tastes incline towards a back alley quickie

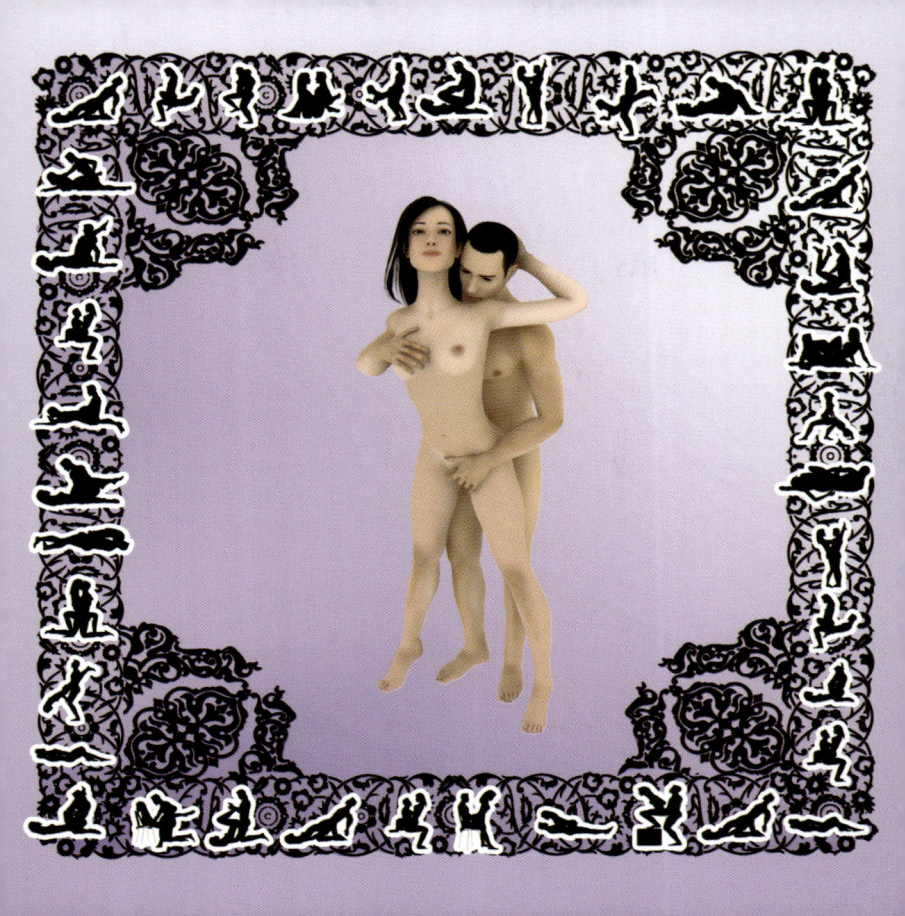

29. THE STANDARD CARRY

The primal response to the overwhelming urge to have sex right here, right now. The man supports the woman by holding her buttocks while the woman clings to his neck. Using his legs for leverage, she can clench her thighs together to narrow the vaginal canal. Not suitable for men with back problems, or couples where the woman is heavy.

DIFFICULTY

● ● ○

Best for: strong, athletic couples who've been swept away by the moment

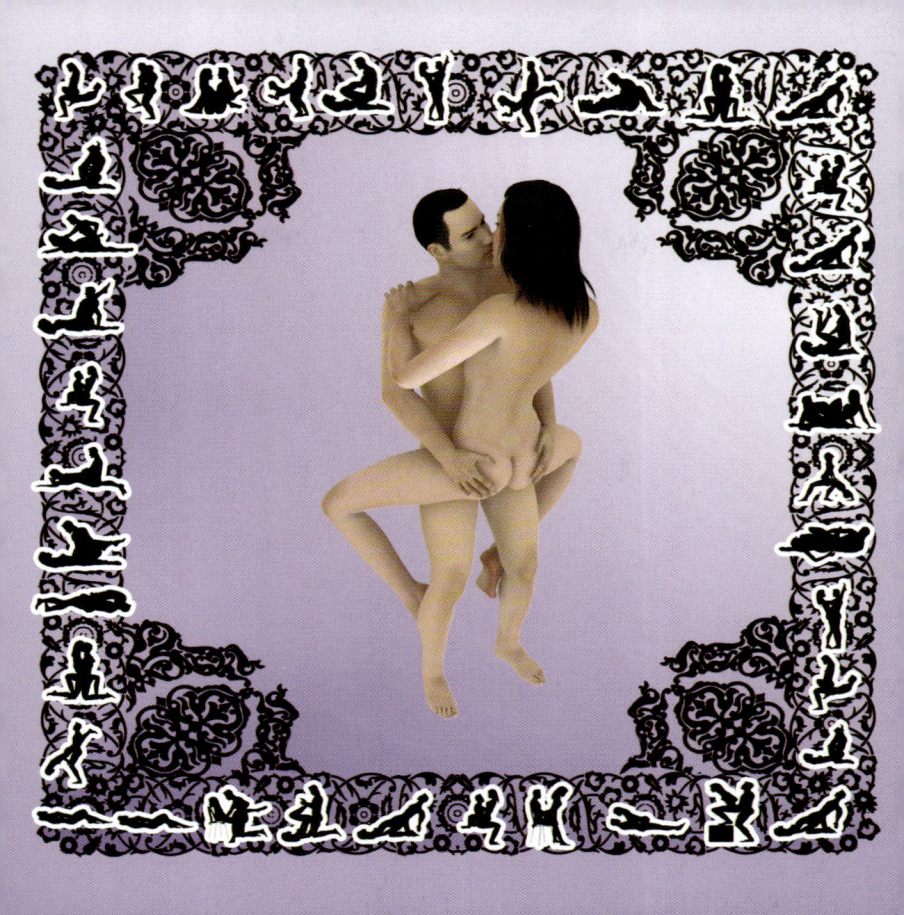

30. THE DANCER

Also known as the Ballet Dancer. This position is ideally suited for those times when you just can't wait to get naked. Facing each other, the woman raises a leg, wrapping it around the man's upper thigh and allowing her to pull him deeper into her. For the flexible, the leg can be raised over the shoulder.

DIFFICULTY

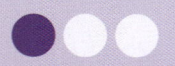

● ○ ○

DIFFICULTY IF THE LEG IS RAISED OVER THE SHOULDER

● ● ●

Best for: spontaneous or outdoor sex and couples who are a similar height to each other

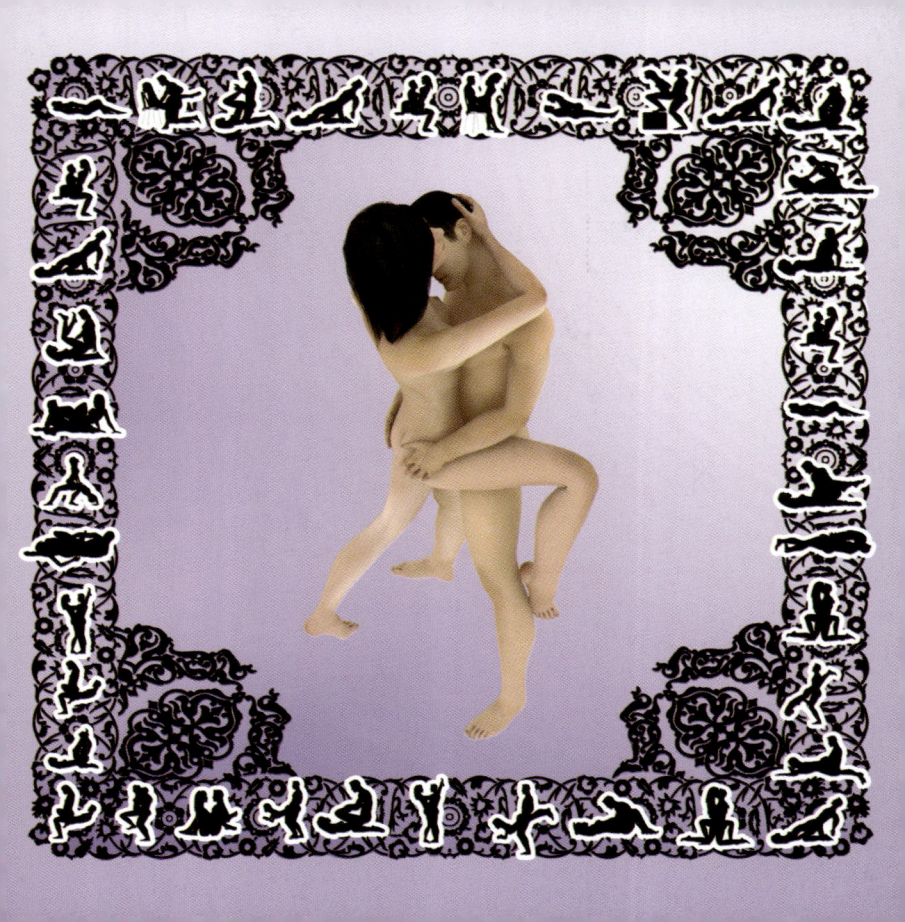

31. THE FIRE HYDRANT

The woman kneels, using a chair for support. The man kneels behind her, raising one of her legs and placing it on his knee before entering her. Changing the angle of the leg will affect the angle of penetration and so should be experimented with – the results will be hot!

DIFFICULTY

● ● ○

Best for: shallow or deep penetration, depending on your mood

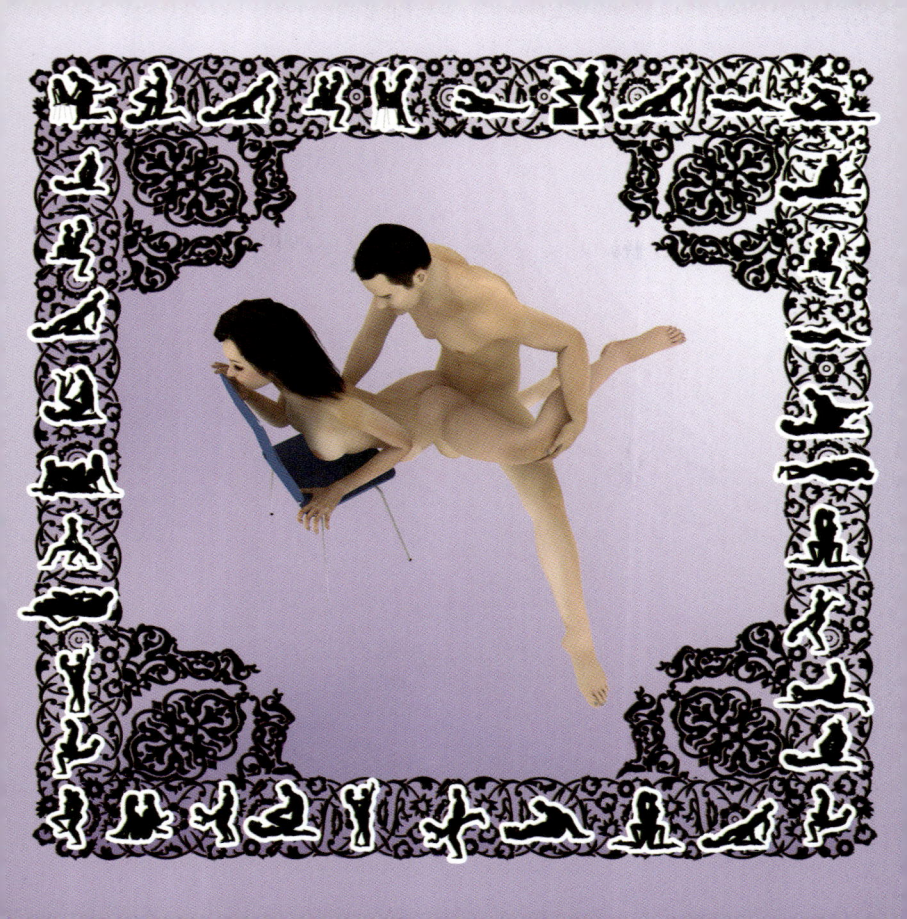

32. SIDEWINDER

The woman lies on her side, facing slightly down. The man, in a kneeling position, enters from behind. Raising the woman's free leg and supporting it with his hand allows a great deal of control for the man without her having to support his weight.

DIFFICULTY
● ● ○

Best for: couples where the man is on the heavy side

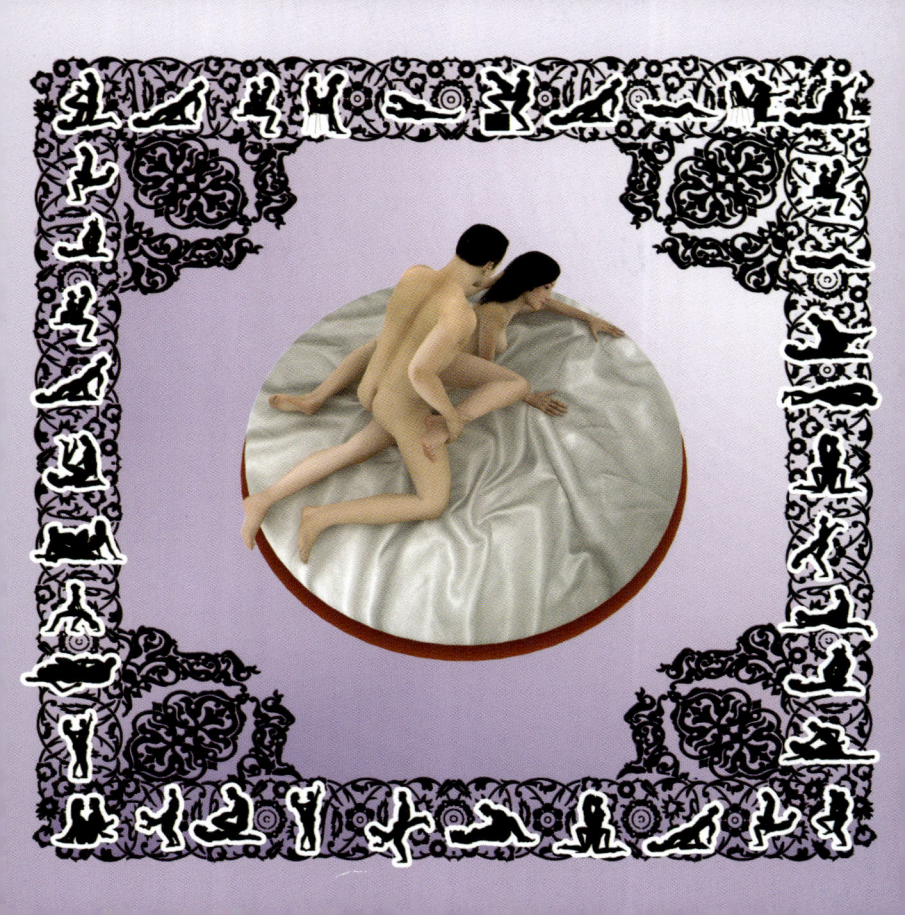

33. THE VISITOR

Like the Dancer, this is another position that's perfect for sex anywhere, any time. Standing face to face, the man stimulates his partner's genitals with his penis, then penetrates her. This works best if the couple are of a similar height, but if not, she can wear high heels, or stand on a low stool.

DIFFICULTY

●○○

Best for: acting on spontaneous desire, as no preparation is necessary

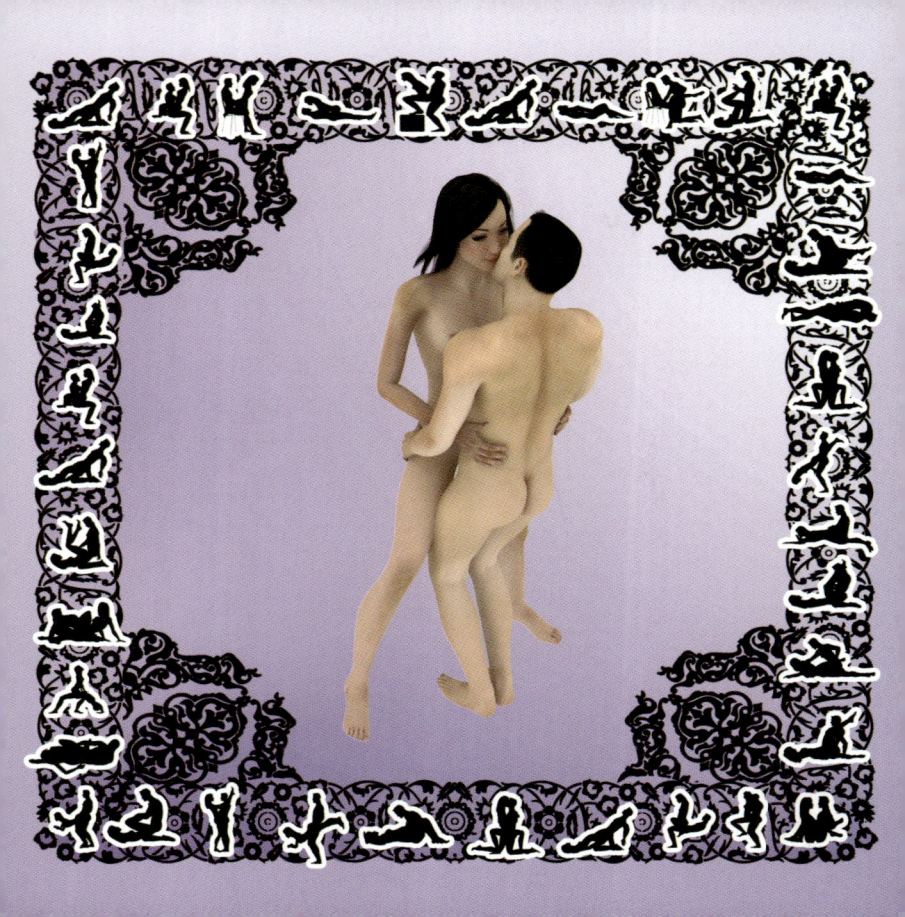

34. THE ASCENT TO DESIRE

The man stands with his feet firmly on the ground, hip width apart, knees slightly bent. The woman stands before him. As he lifts her onto him, she wraps her legs around his hips. It may be useful to start off sitting on the bed, then turn round once lifted so she can put her feet down and help support the lifting motion with the edge of the bed. As she moves up and down, the angle of penetration will alter. This position is not recommended for couples where the woman is on the heavy side, or the man has back problems.

DIFFICULTY
● ● ●

Best for: men who lift weights on a regular basis

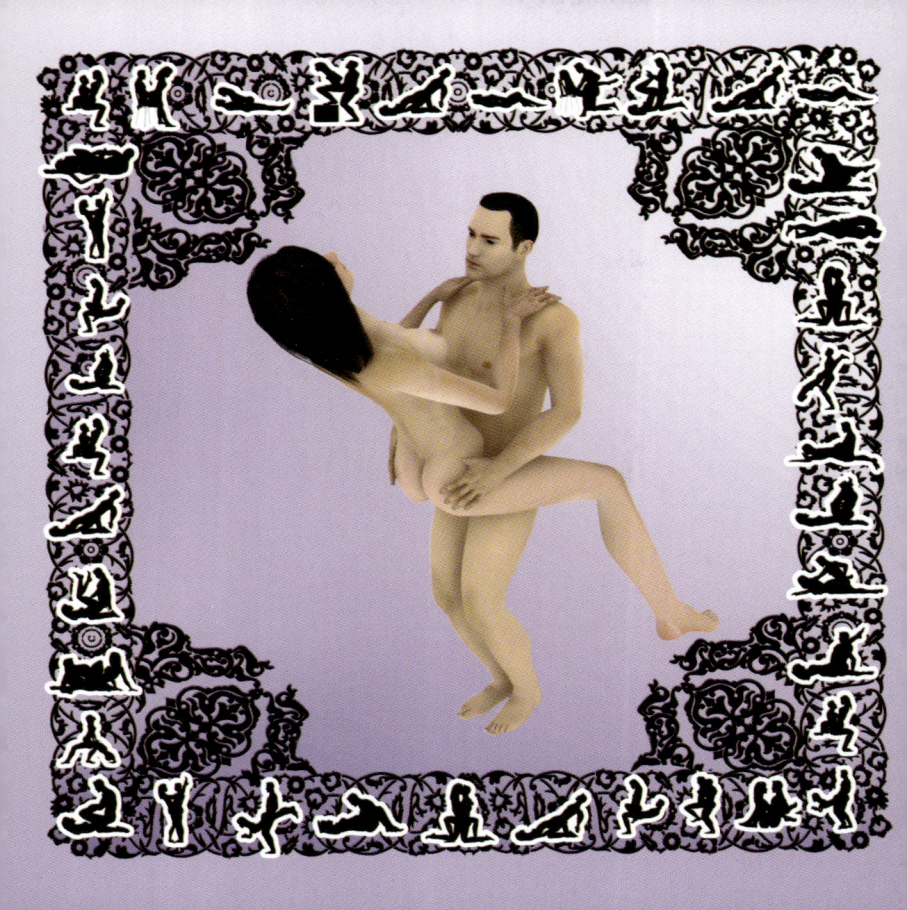

35. THE CURLED ANGEL

A variation on the Spooning Position. The woman curls up on her side, knees drawn up, and the man spoons her from behind. From his position, penetration is fairly easy and he can reach around to play her breasts or clit. This position is especially recommended for pregnant women, as it can be adapted so she doesn't have to bring her knees up quite as far and so avoids squashing her baby bump.

DIFFICULTY
● ● ○

Best for: sex during pregnancy

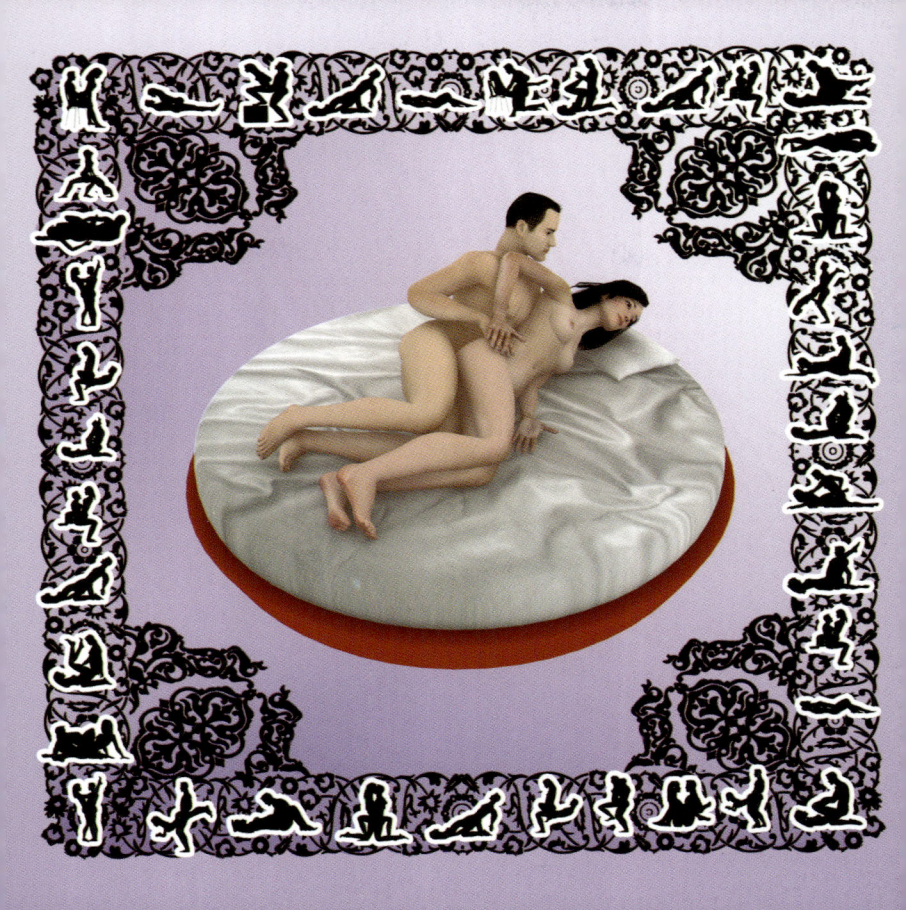

36. THE BRIDGE

One of the hardest positions to adopt for any length of time, the Bridge nevertheless looks incredibly impressive. It should be tried only if the man is very flexible and very strong. He makes a bridge with his body and she straddles him, sitting down onto his penis. Taking the weight on her feet, she then moves up and down on top of him. In this position, the blood will rush to his head, which can increase the intensity of orgasm, but stay in the Bridge too long and there's a definite possibility of passing out.

DIFFICULTY
● ● ●

Best for: show-offs and Olympic gymnasts

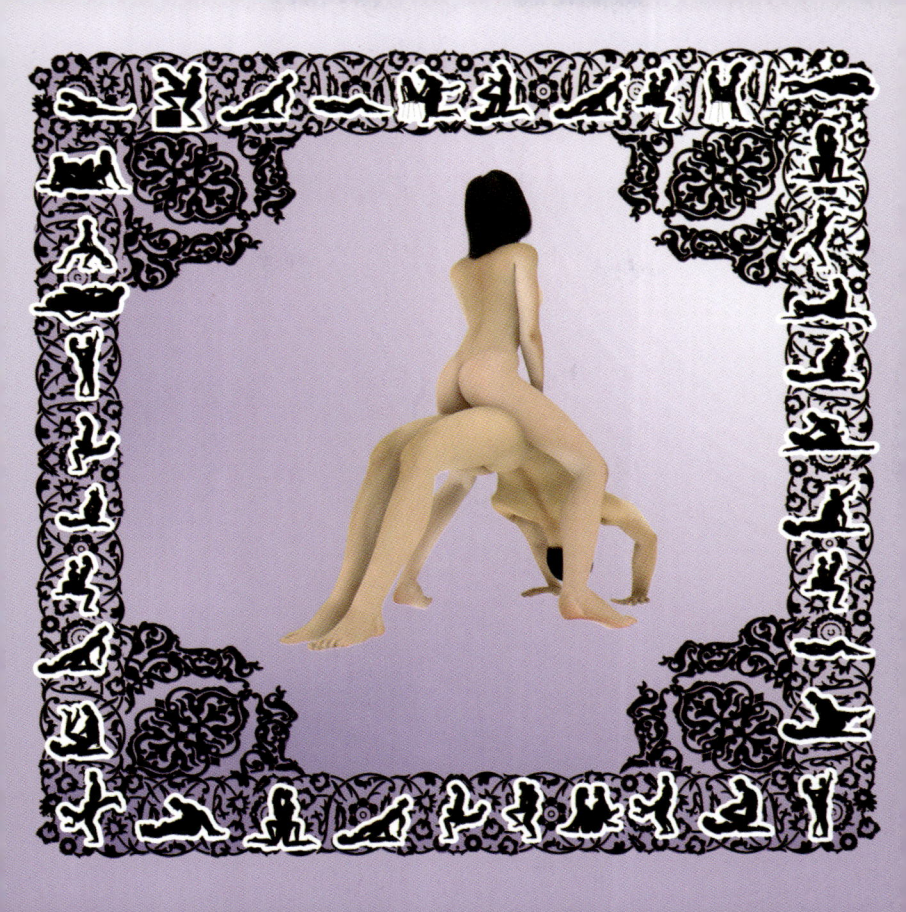

37. THE CLOSE-UP

A variation on simple spooning and the Curled Angel position, but slightly more difficult to master. The man and woman lie on their sides and he spoons her from behind, but this time she wraps her legs around the outside of his. In this position, it's easy for him to stimulate her breasts and clitoris prior to penetration, or she can play with herself while he thrusts into her.

DIFFICULTY

● ● ○

Best for: stimulating her body during sex if she never comes from penetration alone

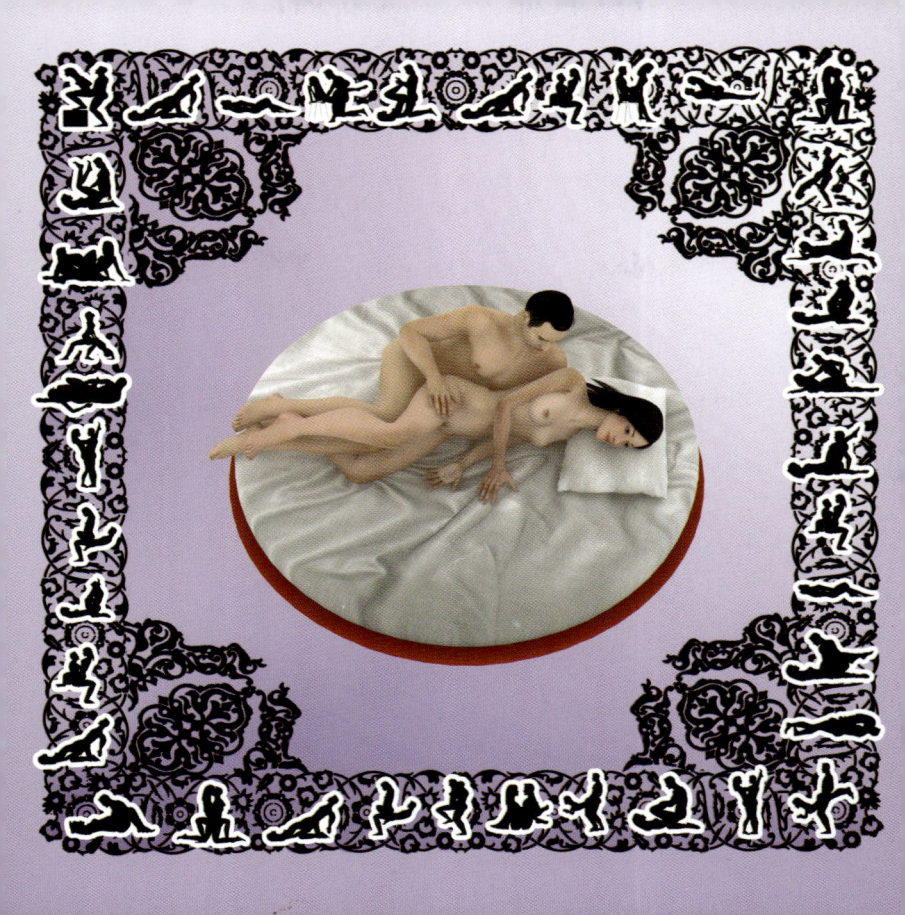

38. THE KNEEL

As its name implies, the man and woman kneel face to face to adopt this position. She straddles his thighs so he can enter her, and wraps her arms around his neck. He embraces her and, moving gently up and down with his knees, penetrates her. This is a lovely, intimate position as it allows for plenty of kissing.

DIFFICULTY

● ● ○

Best for: couples who enjoy close, face-to-face contact during sex

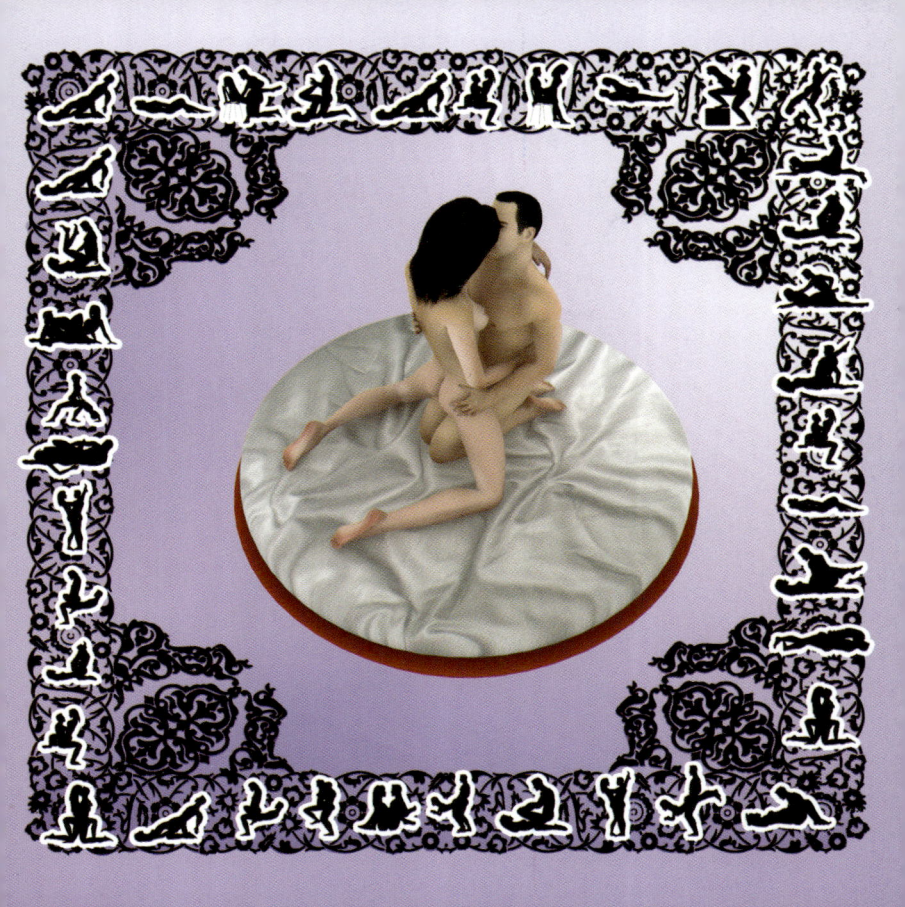

39. THE CROSS

In the Cross position, the woman lies on her back, one leg extended, the other bent up to give her lover ease of access. The man sits down with one thigh over her extended thigh and slips her bent leg under his arm. He can brace himself with his hands behind his back to control the rhythm of the movement.

DIFFICULTY

● ● ●

Best for: allowing him to set the pace of his thrusts

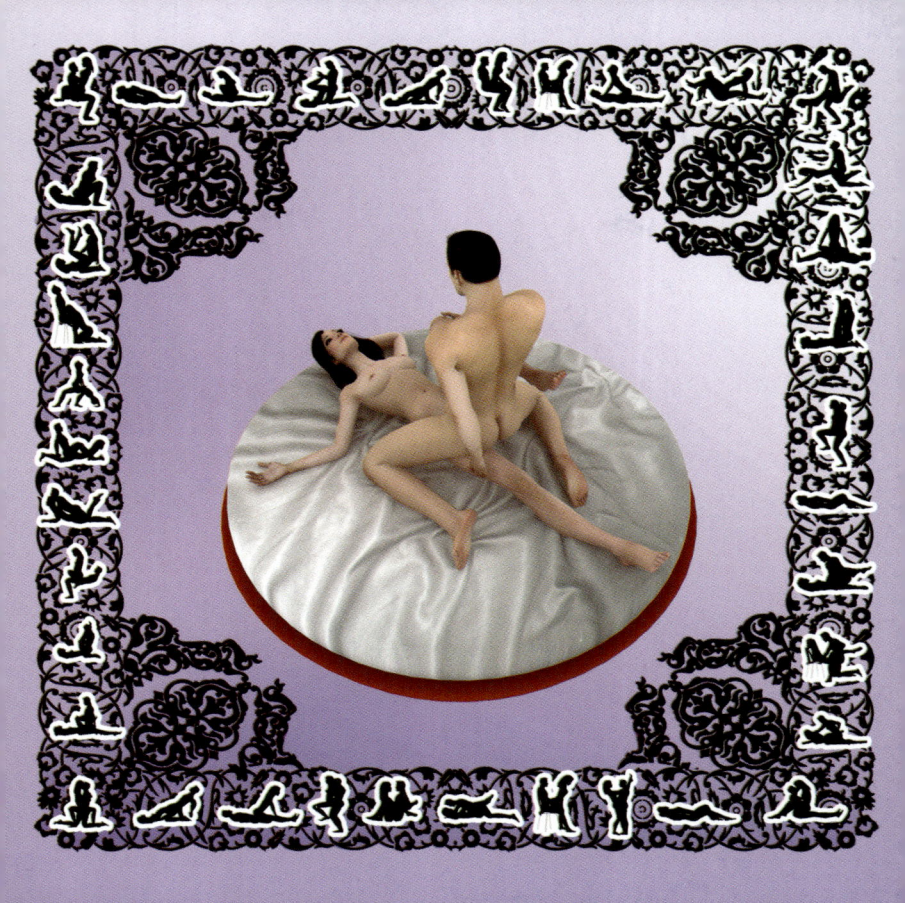

40. THE DECKCHAIR

The man relies on his hands to support his weight in this position, while sitting legs outstretched. With his hands behind him, he leans back, bending slightly at the elbows. The woman lies back, facing him, with a pillow beneath the small of her back for extra support if required, and places her feet on his shoulders. She can then move her hips forward to allow him to enter her.

DIFFICULTY

● ● ○

Best for: really deep penetration

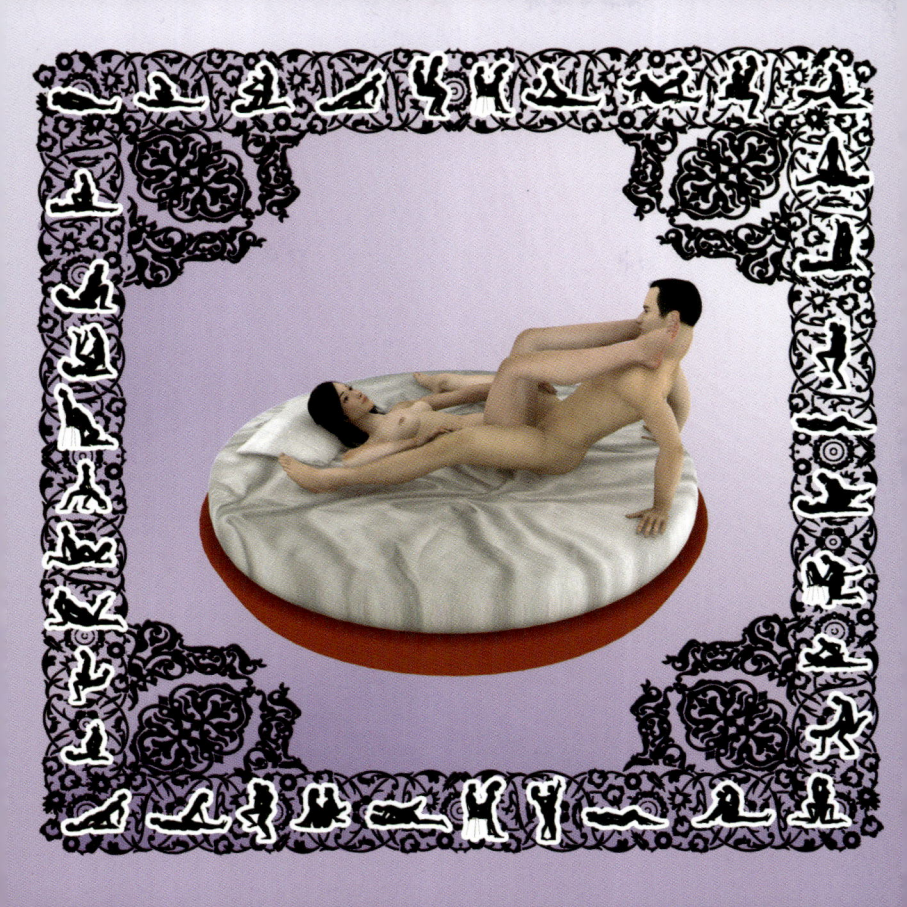

41. THE SQUAT BALANCE

A sex position which requires some skill and a fair amount of strength. The woman stands on the bed or a sturdy piece of furniture, and the man stands behind her. From here, he places his hands on her bottom so she can 'sit' down and lean against his chest. He is now able to penetrate her from behind, while she braces herself on his arms as he supports her weight.

DIFFICULTY

● ● ●

Best for: couples where the woman is petite, as balancing on furniture will ease the height imbalance

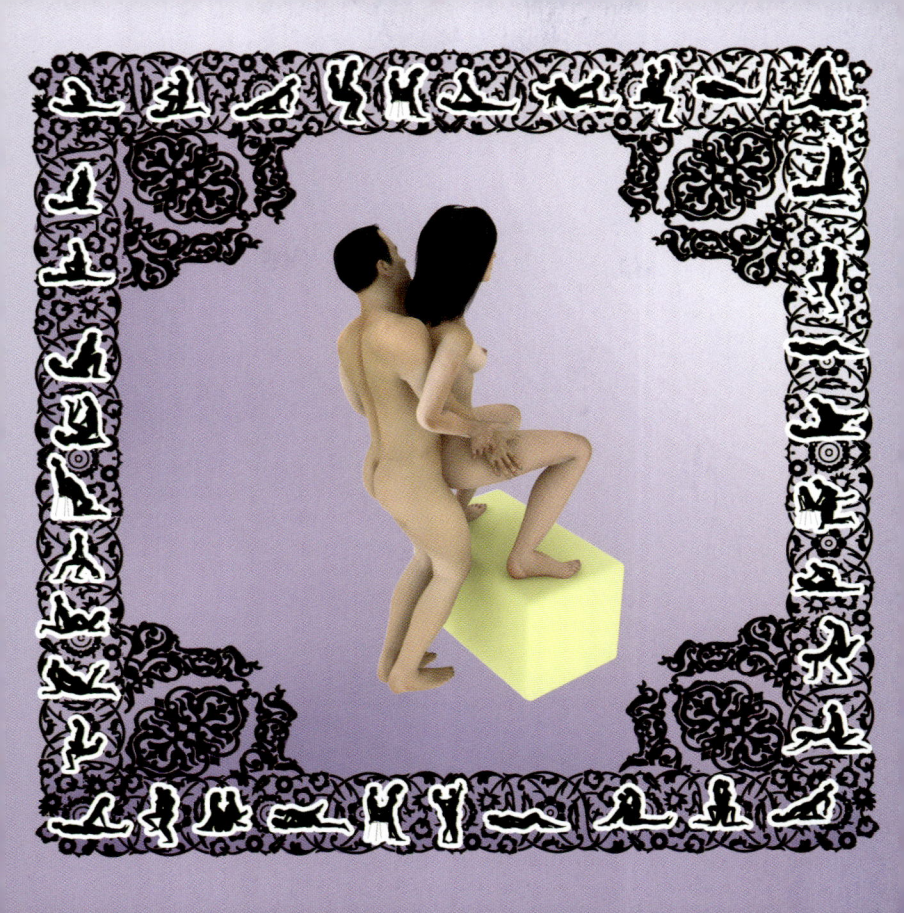

42. THE MAGIC MOUNTAIN

First of all, construct a "mountain" from a pile of pillows, the firmer the better. Once the pillows are at a comfortable height, the woman kneels and leans forward over them. The man kneels behind her, legs on the outside of hers; he then leans down over her and penetrates her from behind.

DIFFICULTY
● ● ○

Best for: people who require extra support during sex

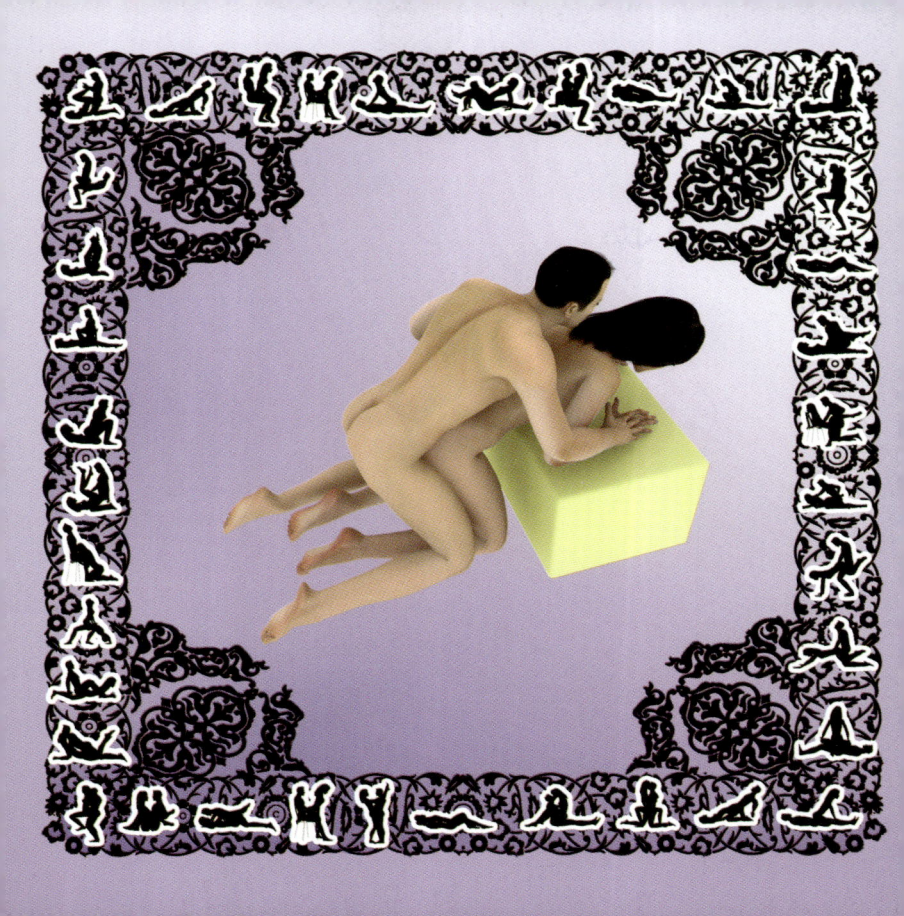

43. THE PROPELLER

The woman lies on her back, legs outstretched and together. The man lies on top of her, with his head facing her feet, as if they're about to get into the 69 position for oral sex. Instead, he penetrates her with his penis, and once he's inside he can make circular motions with his hips. This position may require some practice to get right.

DIFFICULTY
● ● ●

Best for: novelty value, and little else

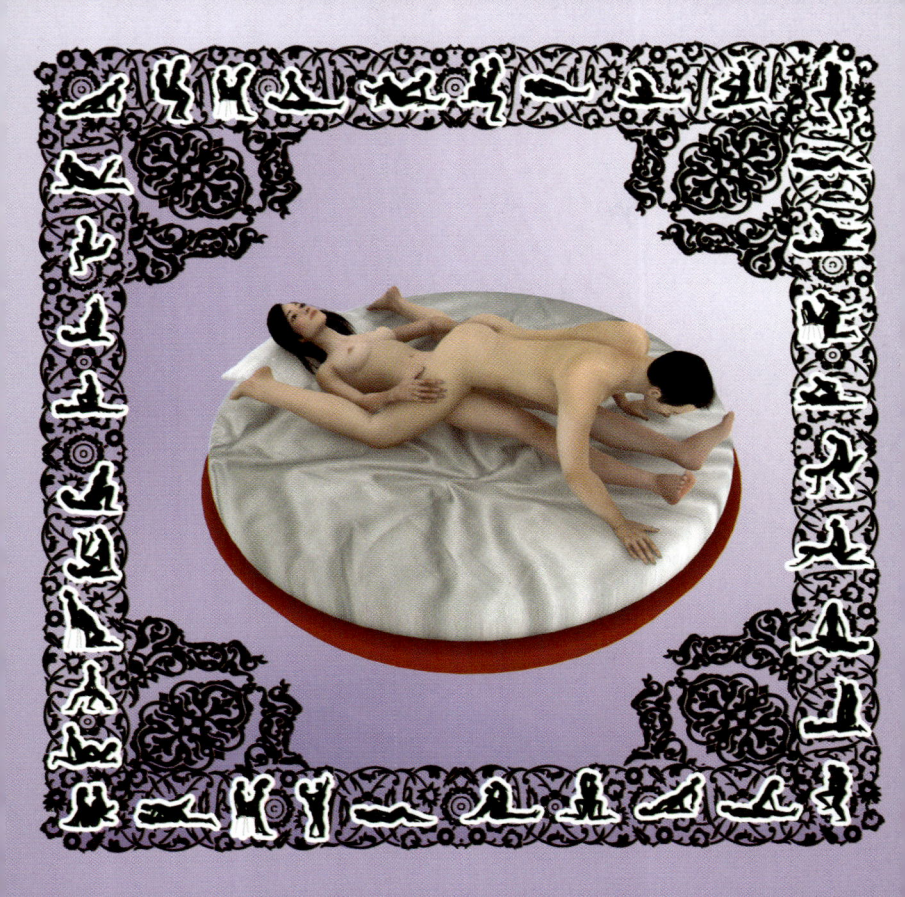

44. THE CROSSED KEYS

The woman lies with her bottom near the edge of the bed, legs straight up and crossed. The man stands in front of her and uses his hands to cross and uncross her legs while penetrating her.

DIFFICULTY
● ● ○

Best for: Playing erotic peek-a-boo

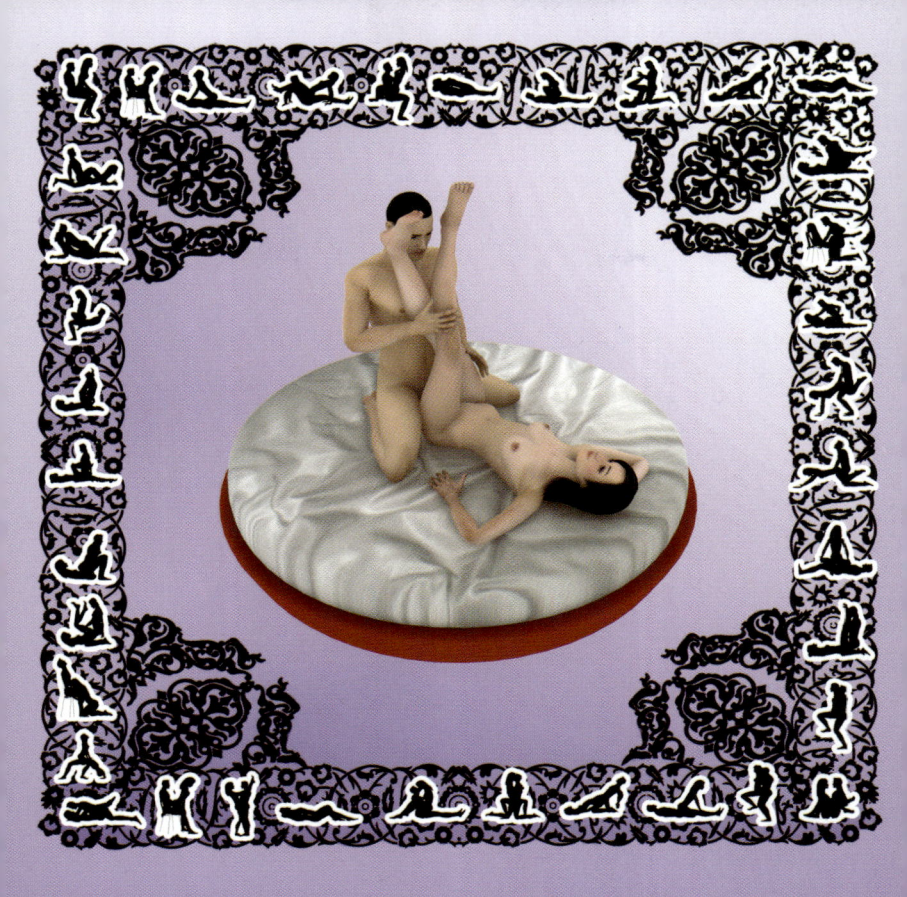

45. THE SHIP

With the man lying on his back, the woman sits down on his groin with both legs to one side, so she's sitting across him like a boat on the water. She is in control of any movement, from a ripple to a tidal wave depending on her mood.

DIFFICULTY
● ○ ○

Best for: letting her take things at her own pace

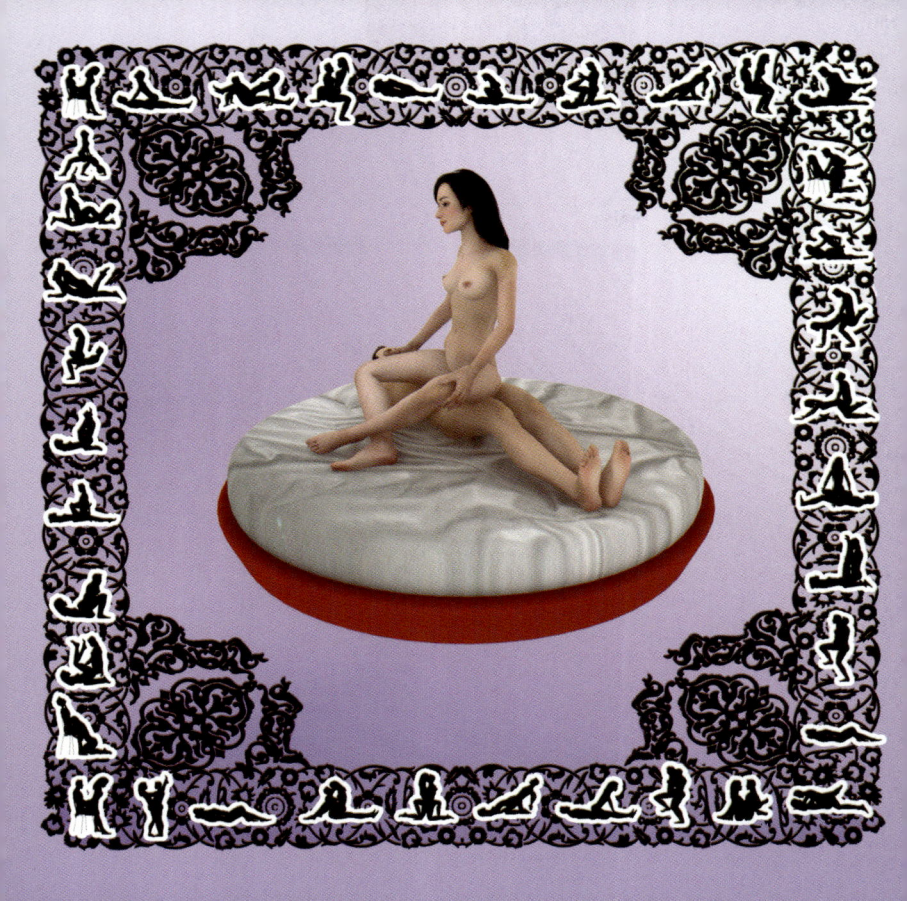

46. THE LANDSLIDE

This position is particularly challenging. The woman lies down on her stomach, propped up on her forearms and with her legs straight and slightly apart. The man sits behind her with his legs in front of him and his hands on either side of his body for support. He leans back at a 45-degree angle to her body so he can penetrate her from behind. As he rocks back and forth, she can bring her legs together so she is gripping his penis more tightly.

DIFFICULTY
● ● ●

Best for: trying a new take on sex from behind

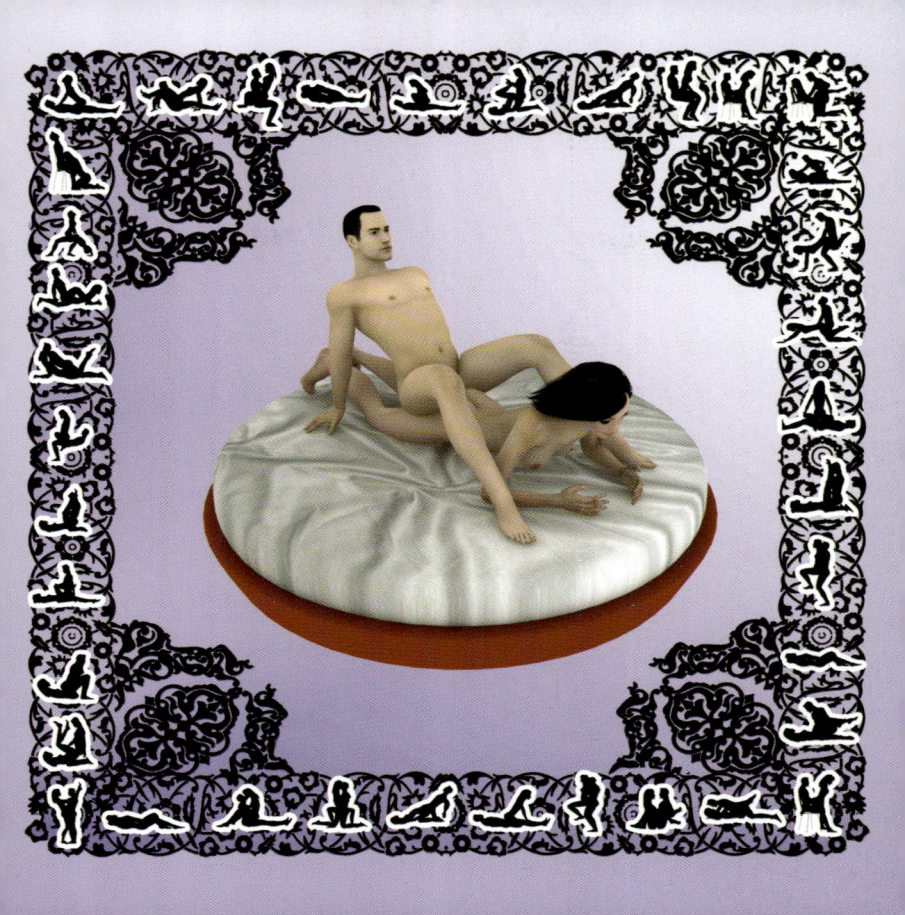

47. THE SLIP

The man kneels up and leans back, taking his weight on his hands behind him. The woman lies back, with her head on a cushion and her back completely flat. She bends her knees either side of his hips to provide the best angle for penetration. Her hands are free to caress her breasts and clitoris as he controls the rhythm and depth of his thrusts.

DIFFICULTY
●●○

Best for: men who want to watch their partner's ecstatic reaction as she is made love to.

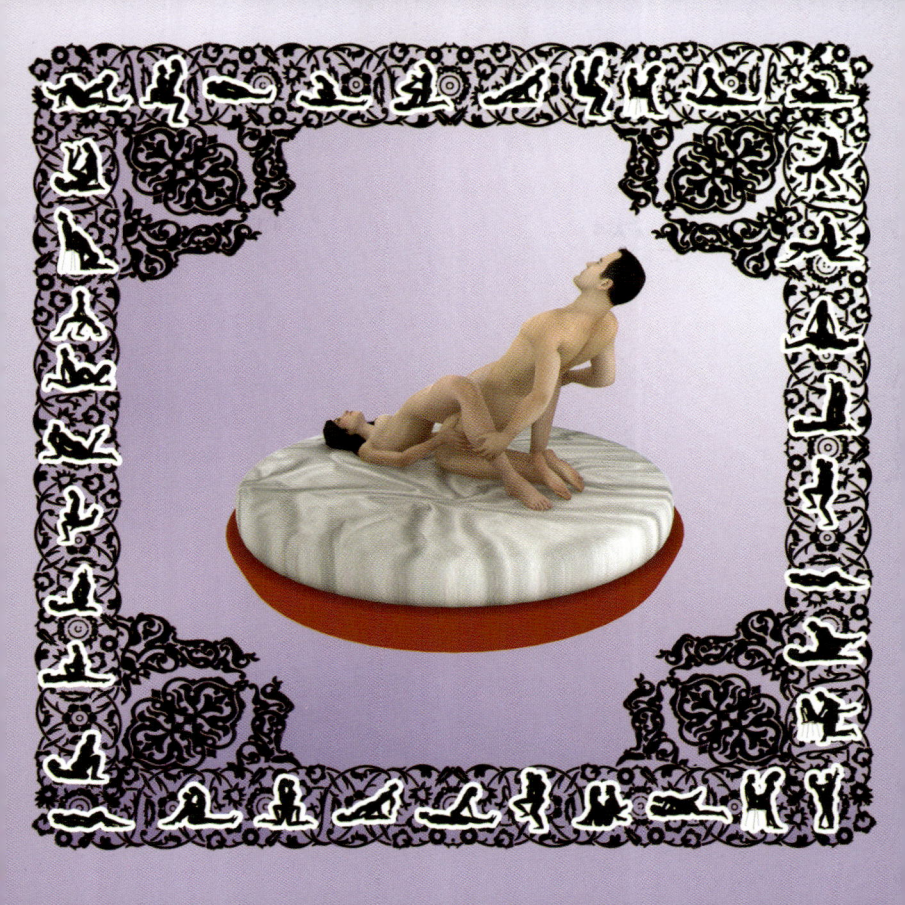

48. THE G-FORCE

The woman lies down on her back and pulls her knees close to her chest. Her partner kneels up in front of her and takes hold of her feet. By thrusting his hips forward, he can penetrate her while controlling the movement and supporting her balance. For even more depth of penetration, she can put her feet on his chest and have him hold onto her hips.

DIFFICULTY

● ● ○

Best for: going just that little bit deeper

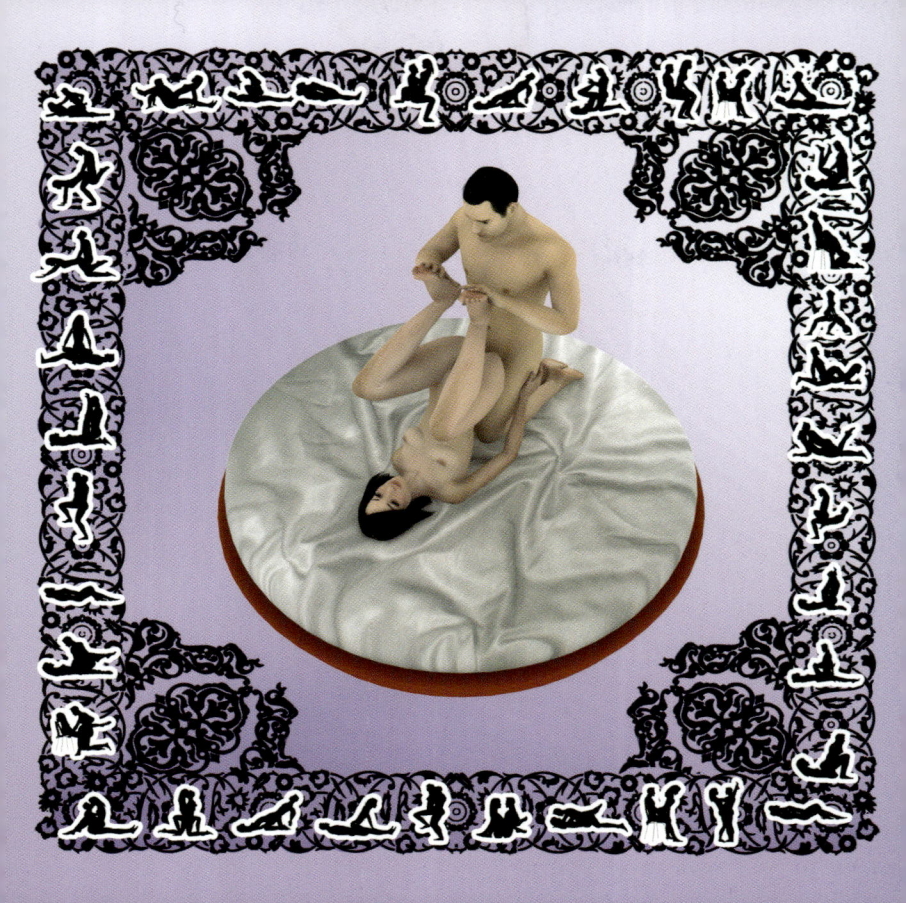

49. THE CHALLENGE

Never was a position more aptly named. This one needs a sturdy chair or other piece of furniture, plenty of flexibility and a great deal of strength. The woman leans forward in a sitting position, with her feet on seat of the chair and her elbows on her knees. The man enters her from behind and takes a firm hold of her waist to help her maintain her balance.

DIFFICULTY
● ● ●

Best for: those who really like to test themselves to the limit

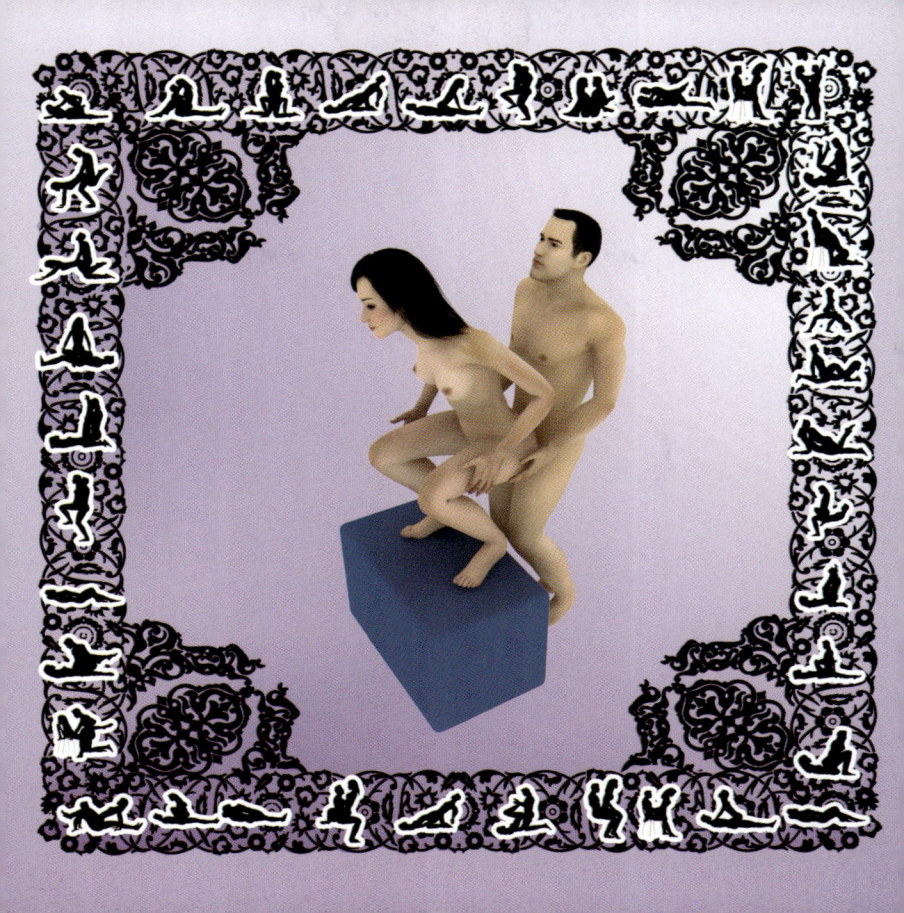

50. THE PEG

The man lies down on the bed with his legs outstretched. The woman then gets on top of him and lets him enter her. As he does so, she stretches her legs out straight behind her and starts to move back and forth at whatever speed she likes. This is an excellent position for full body contact, allowing kissing and caressing throughout.

DIFFICULTY

● ● ○

Best for: well-endowed men, as the position only allows for shallow penetration

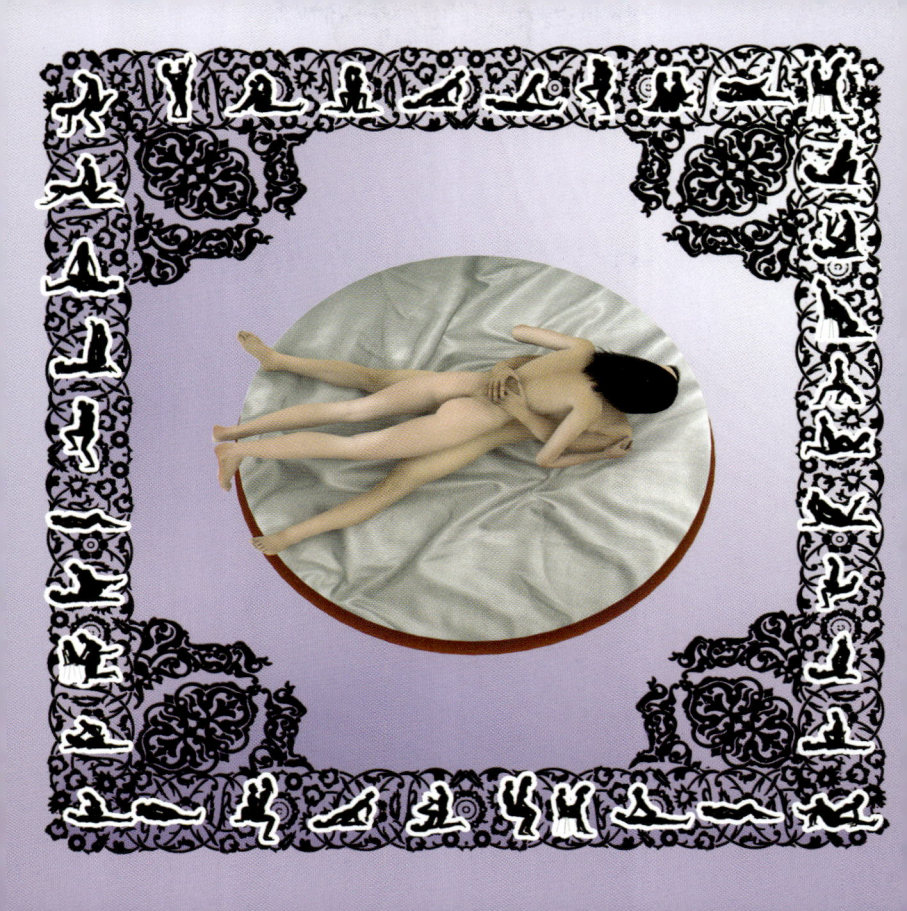

51. THE PROPOSAL

Kneeling face to face, the man puts his left foot flat on the ground in front of him, as though he is proposing marriage, and the woman puts her right foot on the ground and moves close up to him. Penetration can be made by leaning forward towards the planted feet. Any movement in this position is, by its nature, shallow and upright.

DIFFICULTY
● ● ●

Best for: when you've got time for a slow, comfortable screw

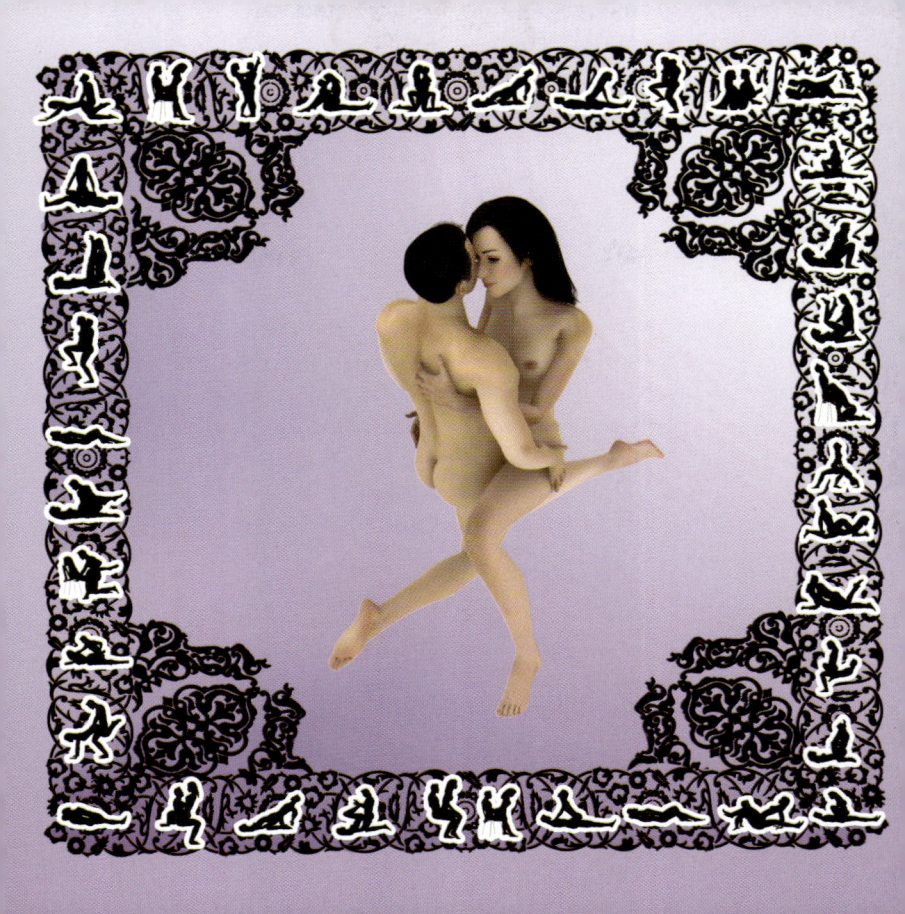

52. THE STANDING WHEELBARROW

In the most challenging of the wheelbarrow positions, the woman starts on all fours resting her forearms on pillows. He kneels behind her to enter her, with one knee bent up and his foot flat in front of him so he can rise to his feet easily. Once he has penetrated her, he reaches down to hold her feet and slowly lifts her as he stands up, keeping his knees bent.

DIFFICULTY
● ● ●

Best for: couples with strength and stamina, as this position is difficult to maintain for long periods

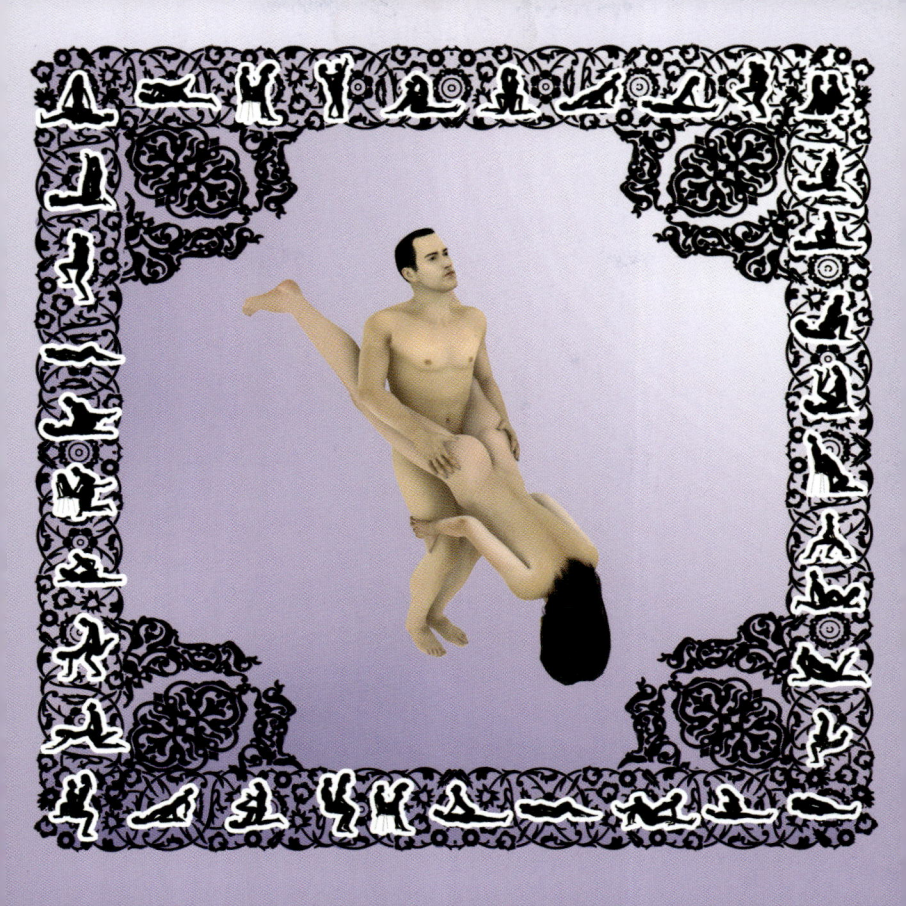

53. THE PRONE TIGER

The man sits up on the bed so that his legs are extended horizontally toward the foot of the bed. The woman turns around and straddles him, with her back toward him, then lowers herself onto his penis. She extends her legs back so they are almost behind her lover, relaxing her torso onto the bed between his feet. She slides up and down and uses his feet for leverage.

DIFFICULTY

● ● ●

Best for: men who like to caress their partner's bottom during sex

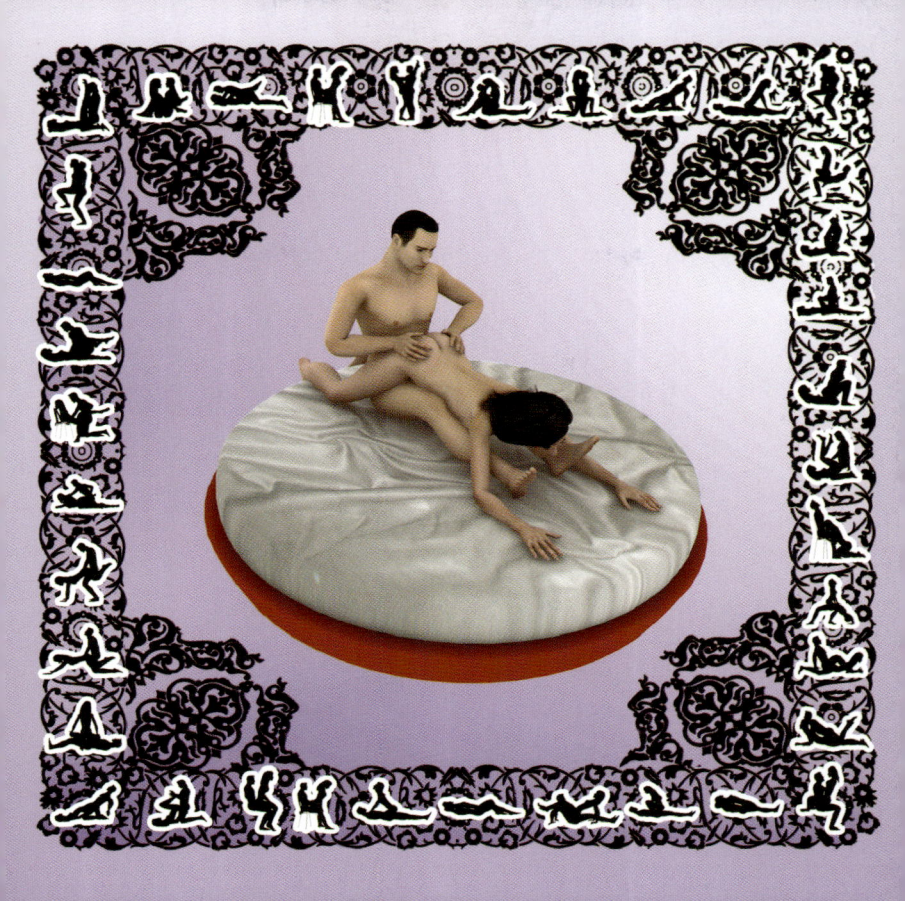

54. THE YAWNING

The woman lies on her back, legs raised and wide open. Her lover leans over her in a dominant posture, resting on his hands and using his thighs to support her. In this position, penetration is deep and intense. He controls the speed of the thrusts, but she can vary the position of one or both legs to alter the sensation, and even wrap them round the small of his back to clench him tight.

DIFFICULTY

● ● ○

Best for: the opportunity to share deep kisses as well as deep penetration

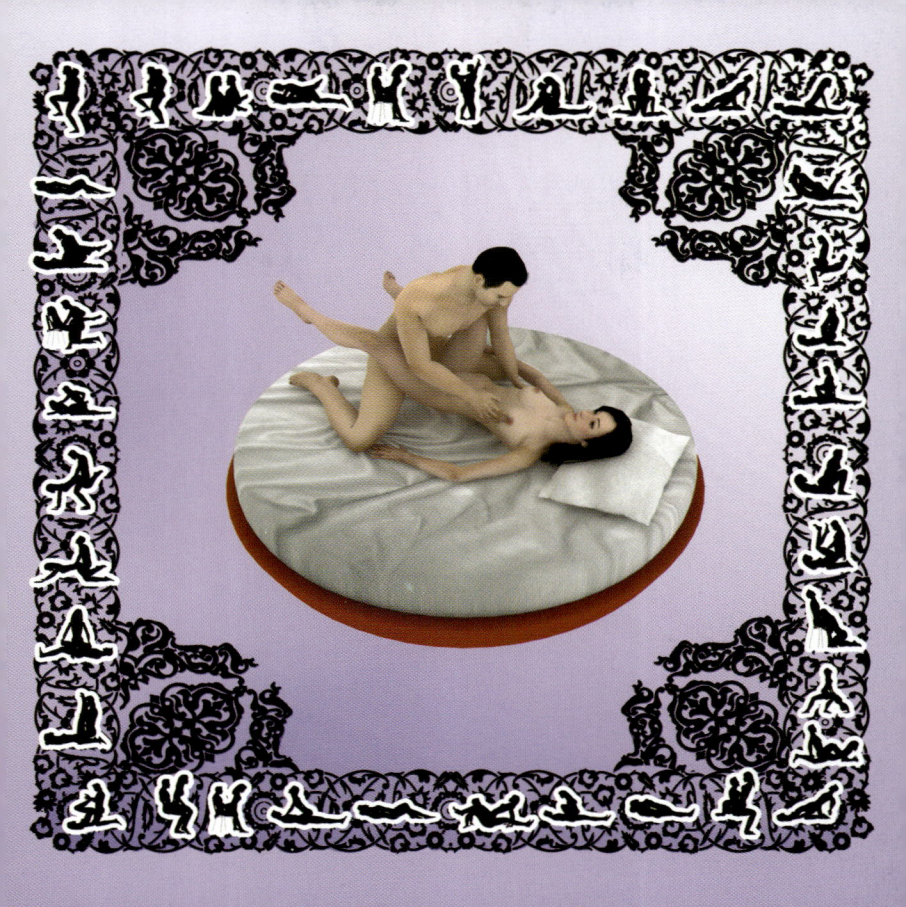

55. THE CRISSCROSS

The woman starts by lying on her side with her arms above her head. The man then lies on his side, his body perpendicular to hers. She raises her top leg so he can slot himself in between her thighs. He holds her shoulders to give himself leverage for a gentle rocking motion.

DIFFICULTY
● ● ●

Best for: slow, shallow penetration

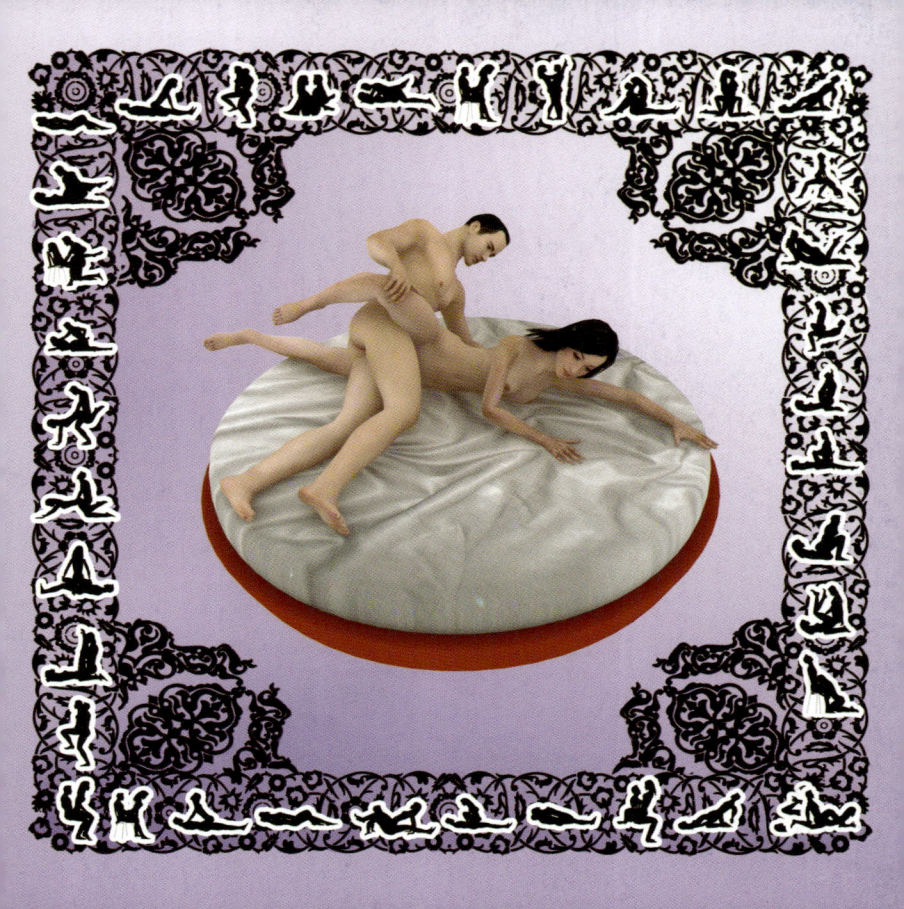

56. SPLITTING THE BAMBOO

In a more athletic variant on the Spooning Position, the man kneels behind the woman, raising her leg up to his shoulder and entering from behind. In this position, she is able to play with her own clitoris, or stroke his penis as it enters and withdraws. For the perfect split the raised leg should be alternated repeatedly, which requires good flexibility and stamina.

DIFFICULTY
● ● ●

Best for: couples with plenty of energy

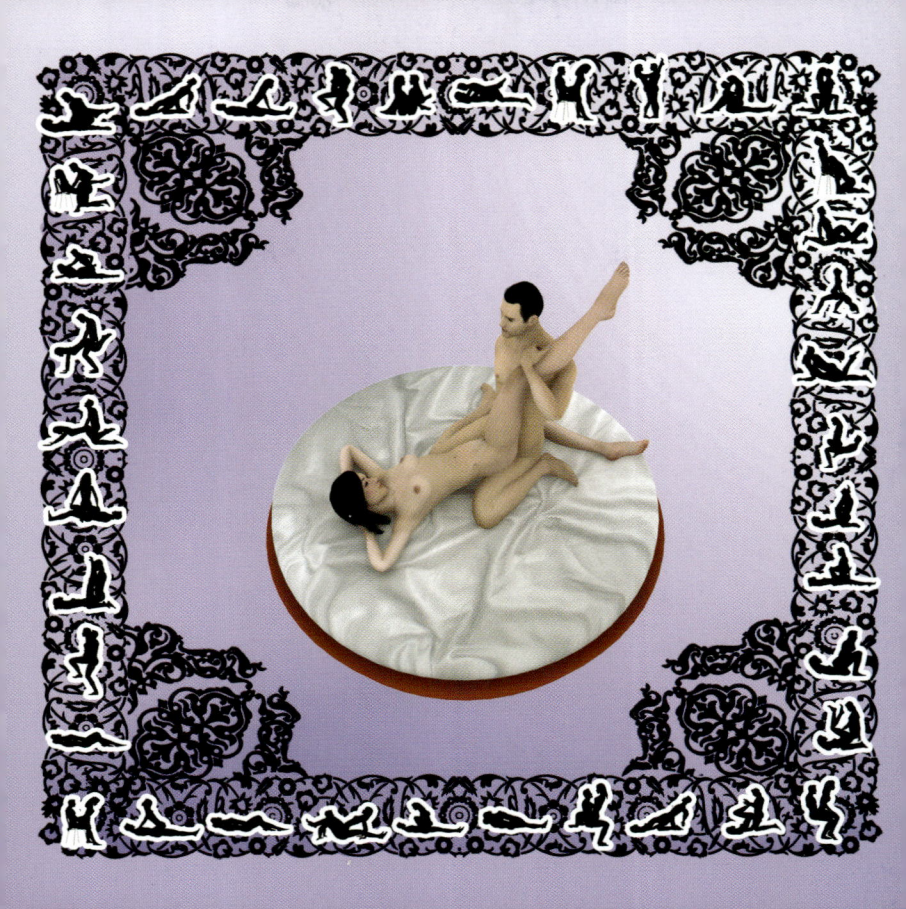

57. THE CROUCHING TIGER

Lying back on the bed with his knees hanging over the edge, the man places his hands on the woman's bottom as she squats over him, facing away from him. In this position, she can reach her clitoris or his balls and penis, and guide the depth and pace of penetration with his help.

DIFFICULTY

● ● ○

Best for: women with plenty of strength in their thighs

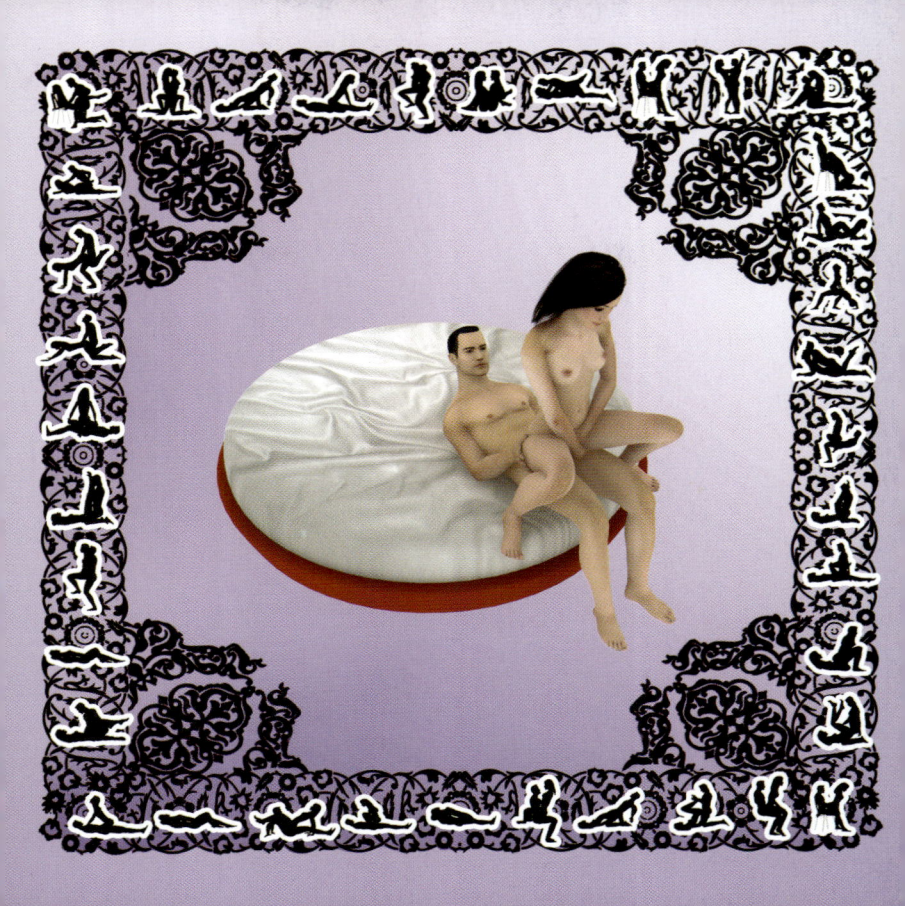

58. THE LUSTFUL LEG

In this position, the couple start approximately shoulder width apart, facing each other. The woman places one leg up on the bed. The man then bends his knees to bring his shoulder under her leg so she can rest her foot on it. She puts her arms around his neck so she can lean back, and he holds onto her hips as he straightens up slowly to penetrate her. She extends her leg and straightens it as much as possible while he gently pushes into her.

DIFFICULTY

● ● ●

Best for: couples with suppleness and stamina

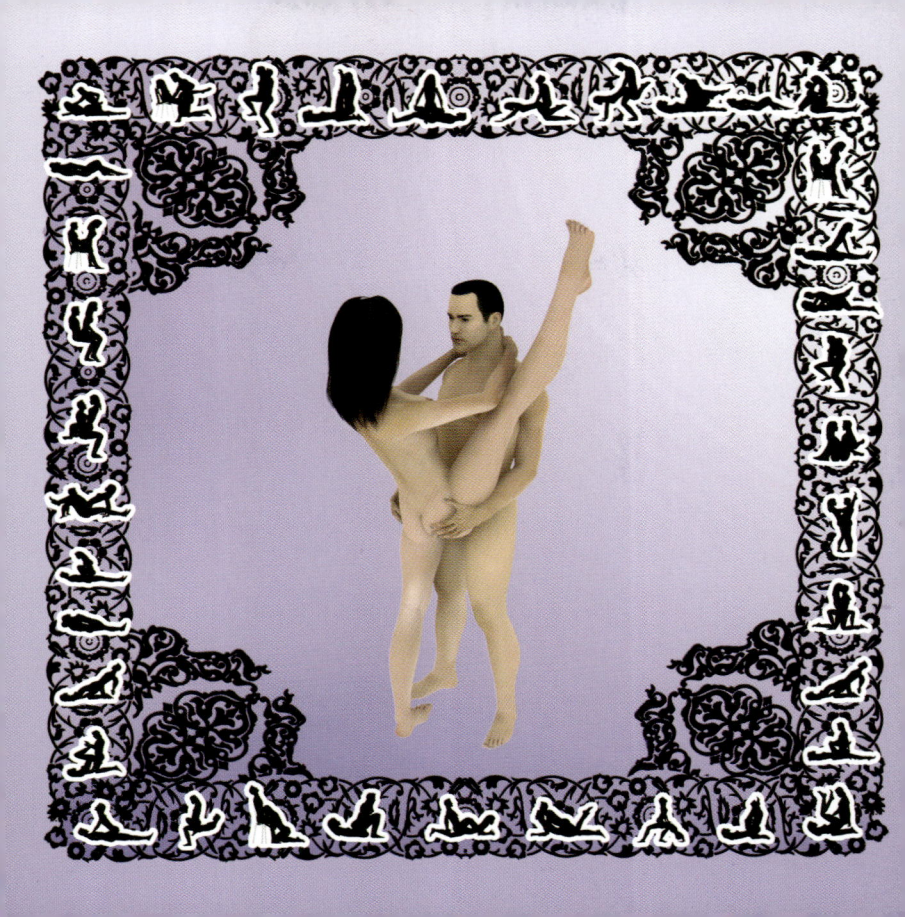

59. THE BANDOLEER

The woman lies on the back with her knees up towards her chest. The man kneels facing her, so she can put her feet on his chest. He leans forward and places his forearms on her knees and she reaches down to grip his thighs. She can increase the depth of penetration by pulling him closer.

DIFFICULTY
● ● ○

Best for: G-spot stimulation: as the man presses her knees down, this stimulation will increase

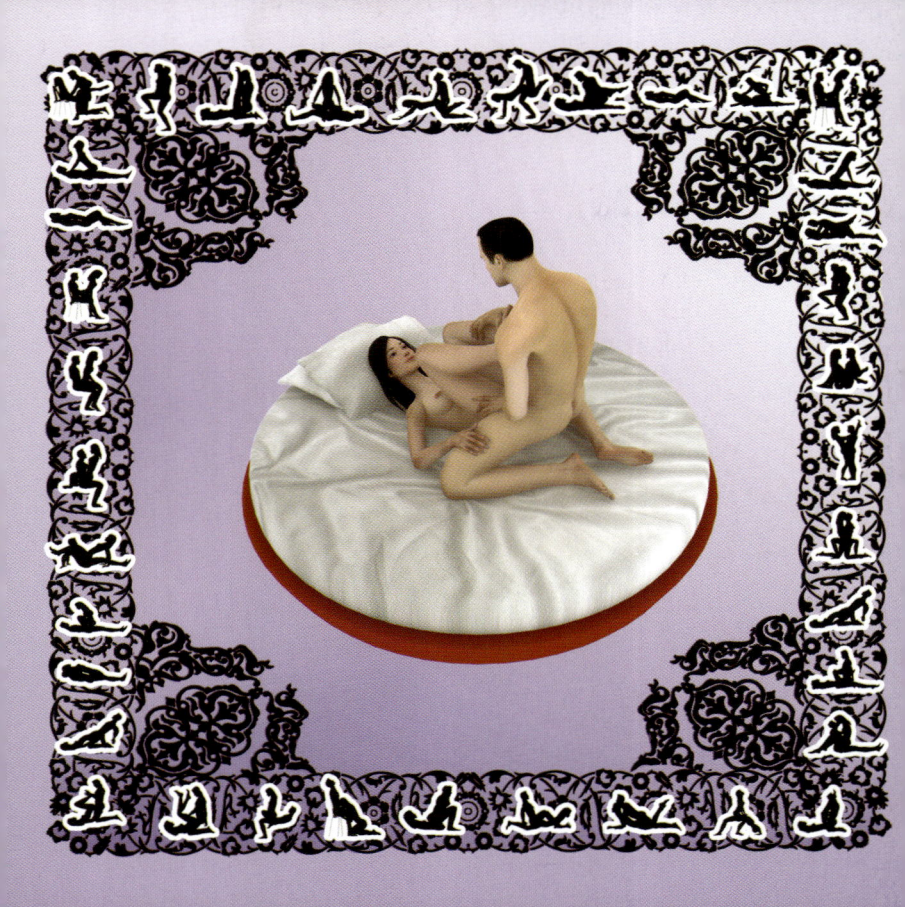

60. AFTERNOON DELIGHT

This is a good position to rest in, tender and romantic. The woman's hands are free for caresses and she can enjoy the intimacy of gazing into her lover's eyes. She lies back and he lies on his side at a right angle to her. She places her knees over his hip to allow gentle penetration.

DIFFICULTY

● ○ ○

Best for: getting the breath back during a long session

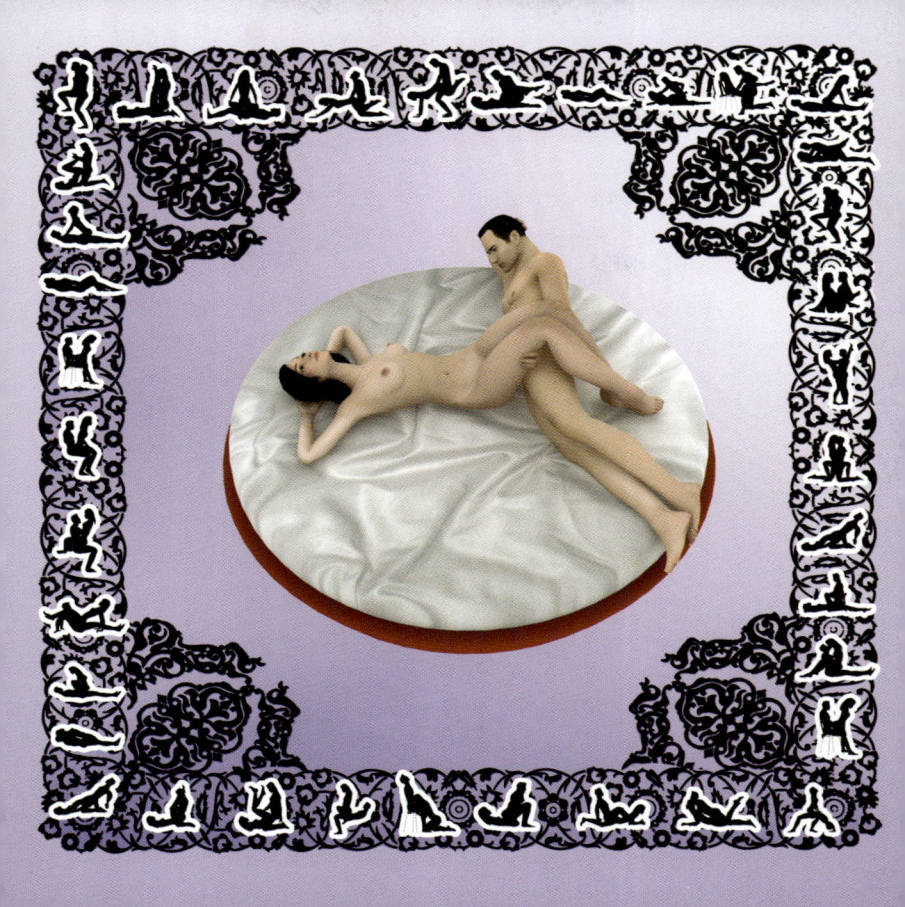

61. THE EAGLE

The man sits on his knees, legs spread, in front of his partner. The woman lies on her back, legs in the air and wide apart. She can relax while he holds her legs up and apart, and in this position he can easily penetrate her with varying speed and depth.

DIFFICULTY

● ● ○

Best for: letting him take control

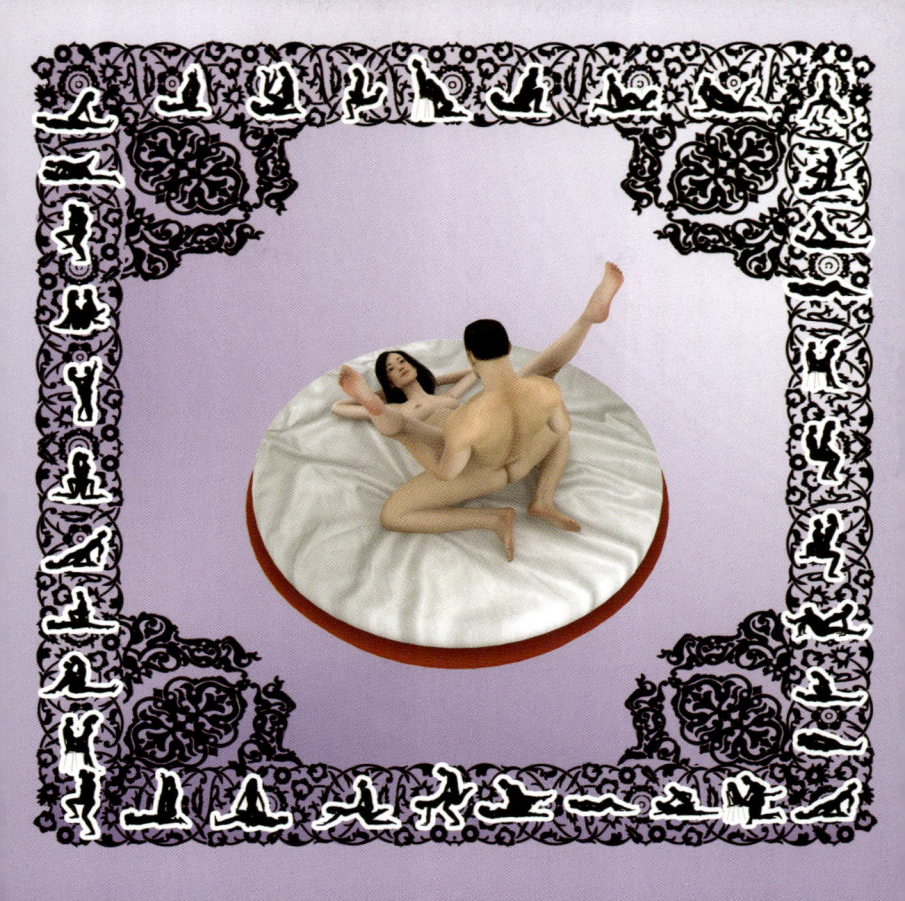

62. THE ROWING BOAT

In this position, the lovers end up clasped together in an intimate caress. The man starts by lying back so the woman can sit down slowly onto his penis. He then sits up, bringing his knees and torso up so the couple are face to face and his knees are on the outside of her body. She should also have her knees bent up so her legs are outside his and she can wrap them around him. He slips his arms over her calves and under her knees, and she slips her hands under his knees and round her thighs so that she can grip his hands.

DIFFICULTY
● ● ●

Best for: slow, gentle penetration and sensual kissing during lovemaking

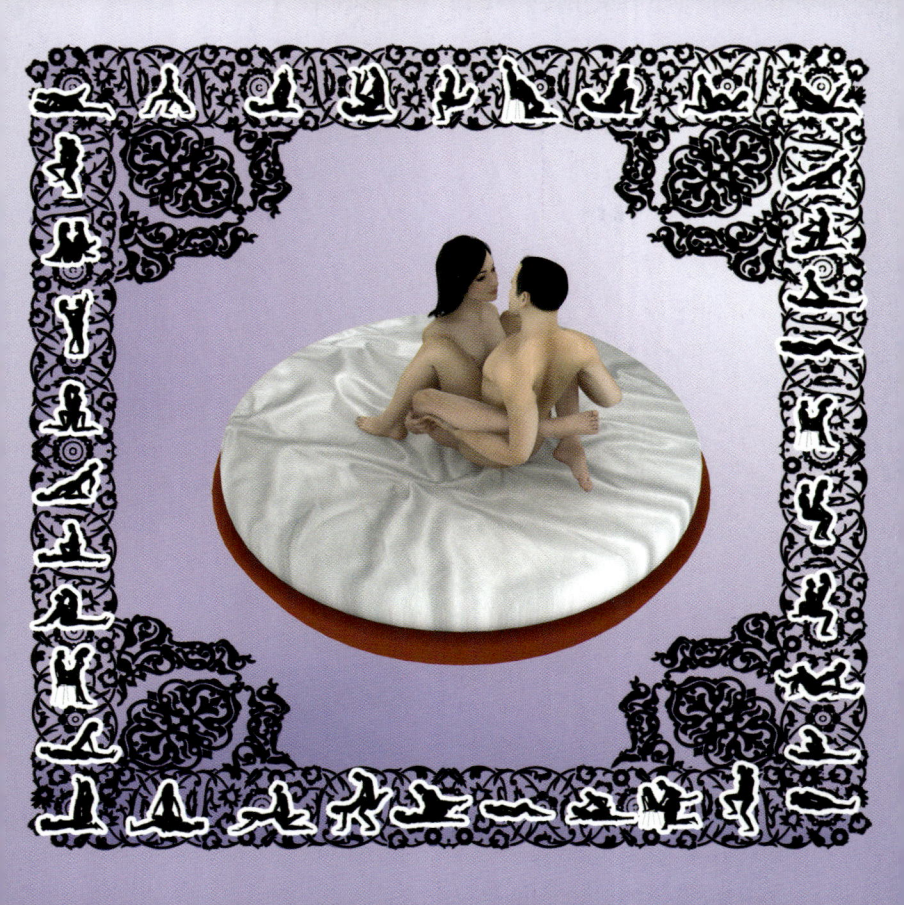

63. THE FAN

The woman stands with her back to her partner. She bends her knees and rests them on the edge of a chair or stool, crossing her arms on the back of the chair or the seat of the stool to support herself. He enters her from behind and controls the movement, caressing her clitoris and breasts with his hands. Penetration will be deep, stimulating the front walls of the vagina and G-spot. This is also a good position for anal penetration.

DIFFICULTY
● ● ○

Best for: anal sex

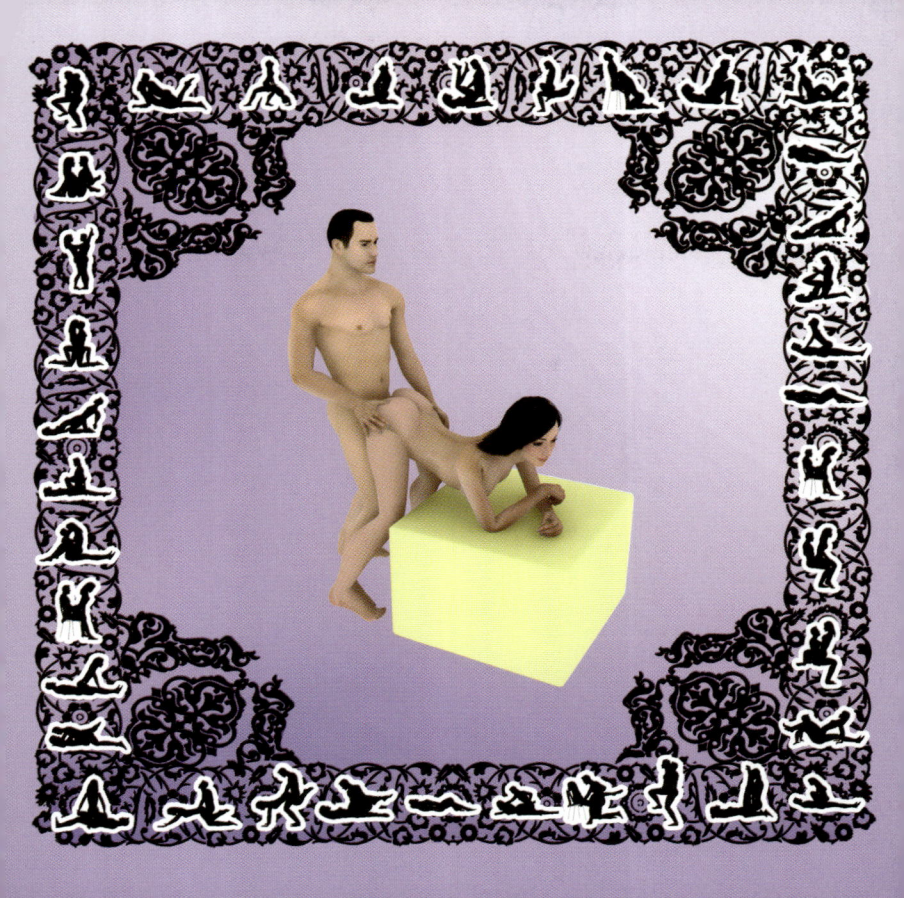

64. THE CRAB

The woman lies on her back and stretches her legs back over her head, as if she is about to perform a backward roll. The man kneels over her, helping her to keep her hips elevated as he penetrates her. Raising her legs in this way helps to shorten and tighten her vagina, so that even shallow thrusts will hit all the right spots, and in this position, he can withdraw to lick her clit before returning to enter her with his penis again.

DIFFICULTY
● ● ○

Best for: when you're in the mood for quick, urgent release

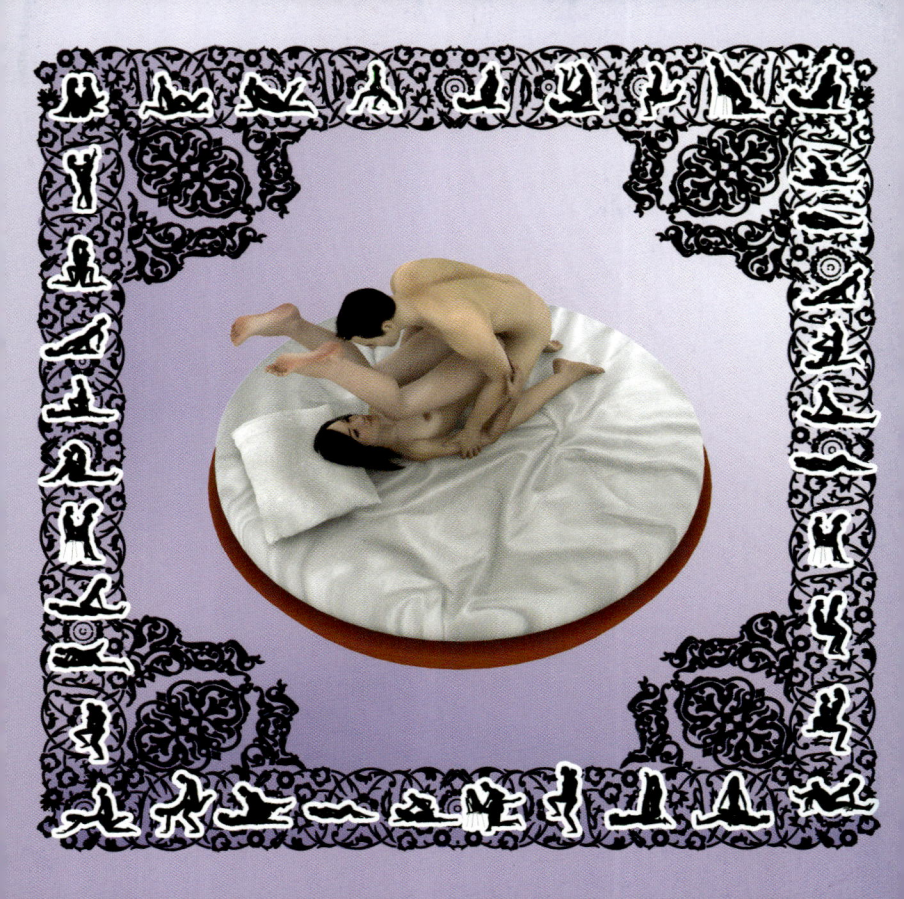

65. THE JOINTER

The man lies on his side. The woman curls up on her side in the opposite direction so that her head is nearer his feet. With her knees drawn up to her chest, she slips her thighs over his, sandwiching his legs. She twines her arms through his legs while he supports himself on his lower elbow and uses his free hand to guide the movement of his penis in and out or to play with her perineum and anus.

DIFFICULTY
● ● ●

Best for: couples who like anal play

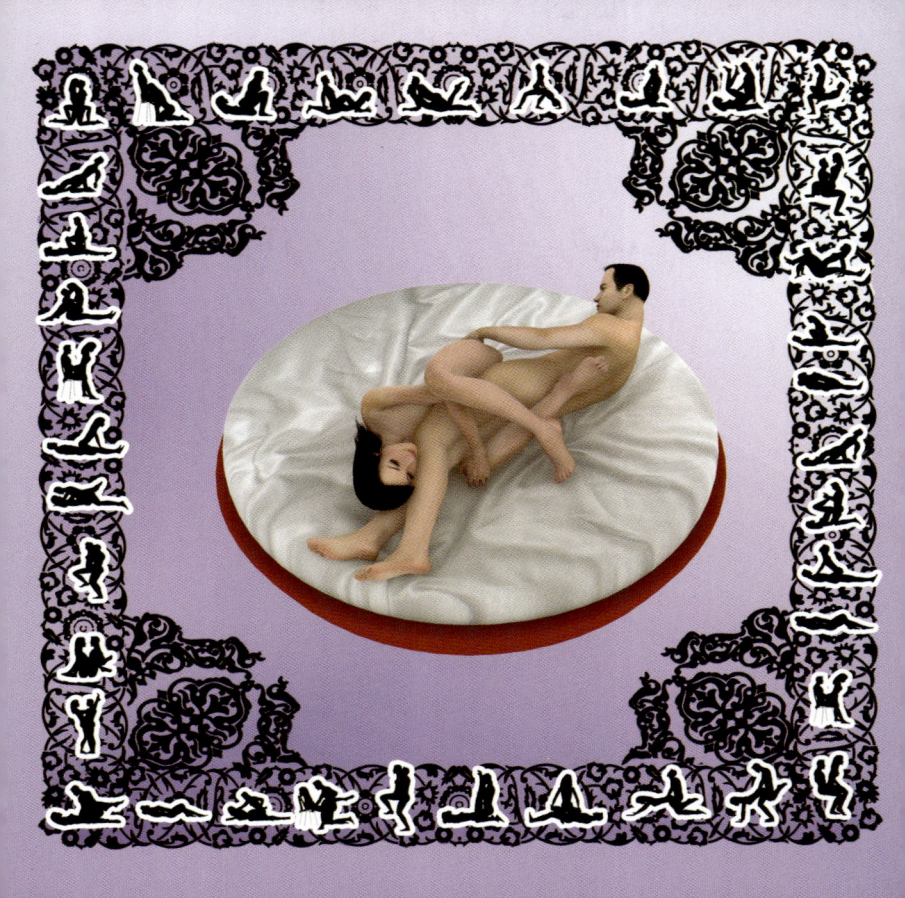

66. THE PLOUGH

The woman lies on the edge of the bed, supporting herself on her elbows. Her legs should be off the bed entirely. The man steps between her legs and lifts her hips and thighs to penetrate her. To perform this position correctly, her legs should be stretched out behind her.

DIFFICULTY ●●○

Best for: deep penetration from behind

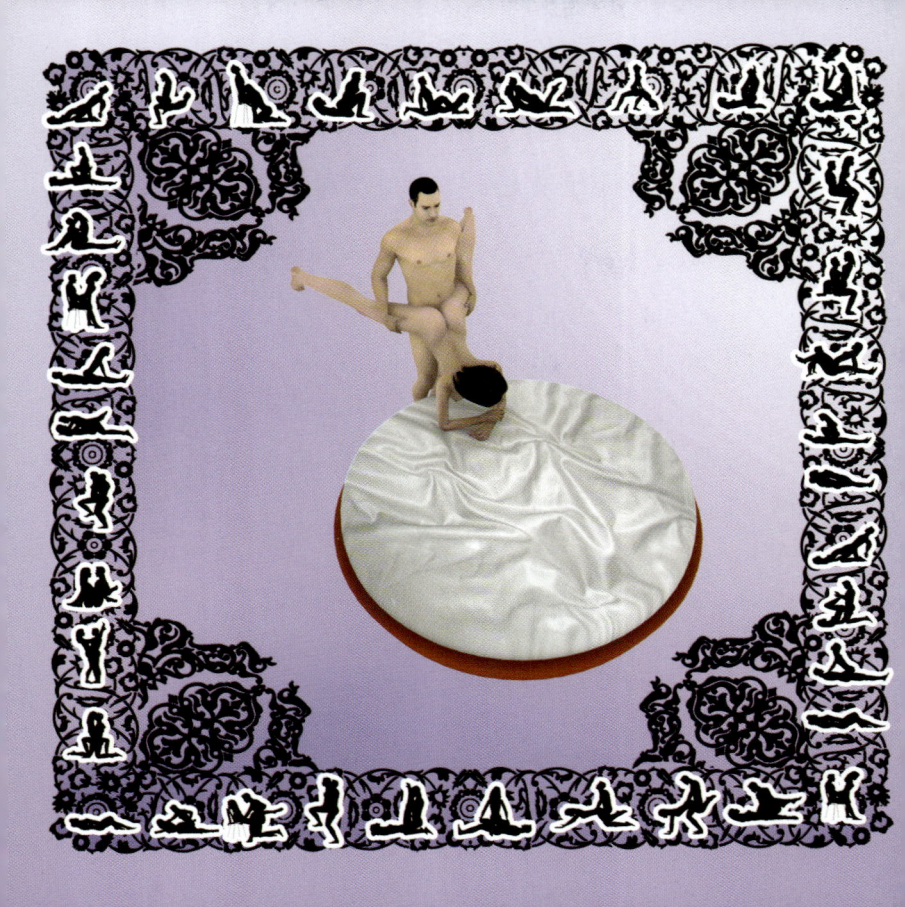

67. THE GLOWING JUNIPER

In this position, the the woman lies on her back with her legs open. The man sits between her knees, facing her with legs outstretched. He lifts her hips to aid penetration and, if he is flexible enough, he can lean down to kiss her belly. Not recommended for men with back problems.

DIFFICULTY
● ● ●

Best for: men who want to display their suppleness

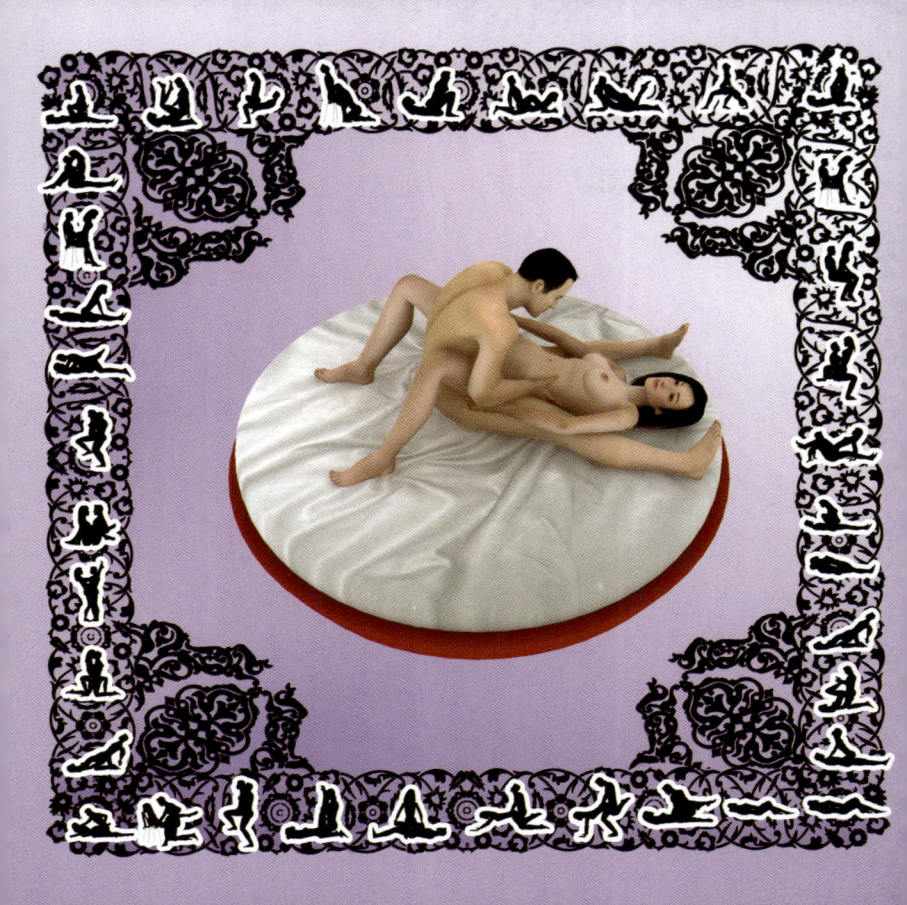

68. THE HERO

The woman lies on her back, pulling her knees up to her chest, feet extended up towards the ceiling. The man kneels on the bed with his thighs under her bottom so she can rest on him as he enters her. He can use his free hands to press her thighs back towards her chest; this will aid penetration and increase the depth of sensation for her.

DIFFICULTY

● ● ○

Best for: offering him control of his movements

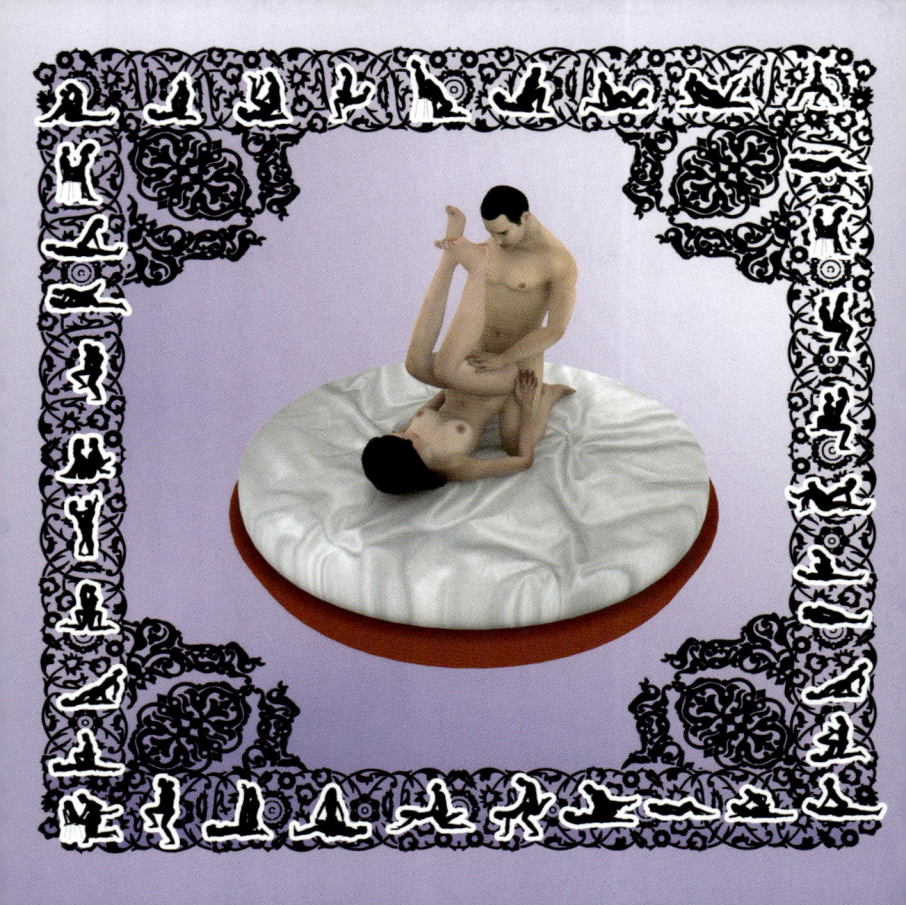

69. THE CATHERINE WHEEL

First the man and the woman sit down opposite each other. Once they're comfortable, she wraps her legs round his torso and he enters her. He then wraps one leg over her to hold her in place. In order to hold her balance, she braces herself with both hands. He guides the movement of his thrusts, propped up on his elbow.

DIFFICULTY
● ● ●

Best for: demonstrating your flexibility

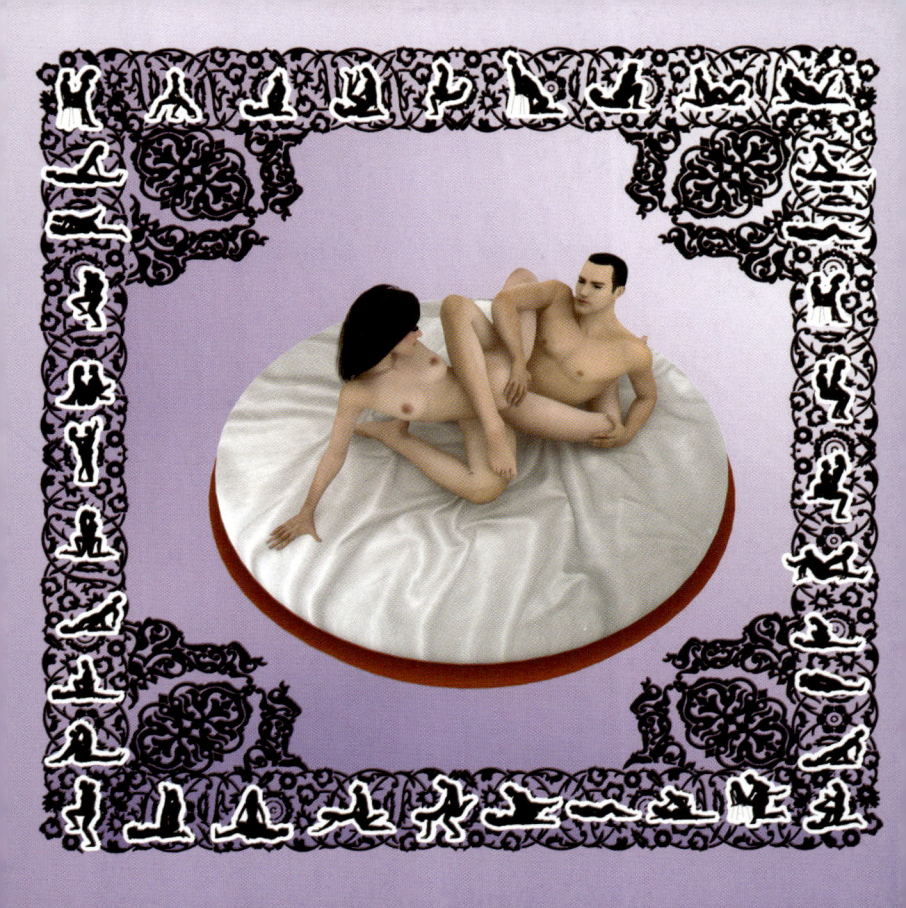

Xcite

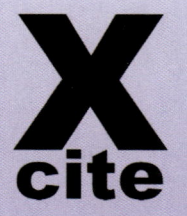

Xcite Books help make loving better with a wide range of erotic books, eBooks and dating sites.

www.xcitebooks.com